Living Translation

Living Translation

Languge and the Search for Resonance in U.S. Chinese Medicine

Sonya E. Pritzker

berghahn
NEW YORK • OXFORD
www.berghahnbooks.com

Published in 2014 by

Berghahn Books

www.berghahnbooks.com

Library of Congress Cataloging-in-Publication Data

Pritzker, Sonya E., author.

Living translation : language and the search for resonance in U.S. Chinese medicine / Sonya E. Pritzker.

p. ; cm.

Includes bibliographical references and index.

ISBN 978-1-78238-310-9 (hardback : alk. paper) — ISBN 978-1-78238-311-6 (ebook)

I. Title.

[DNLM: 1. Medicine, Chinese Traditional—United States. 2. Translating—United States. WB 55.C4]

R601

610.951—dc23

2013033608

British Library Cataloguing in Publication Data

A catalogue record for this book is available from the British Library

Printed on acid-free paper

ISBN: 978-1-78238-310-9 hardback

ISBN: 978-1-78238-311-6 ebook

For my teachers,
including especially my daughter,
Nadya Rose

Contents

Acknowledgments

I have received an enormous amount of support and encouragement over the many years that I have taken to conceptualize, strategize, and enact the ongoing project of thinking through translation in Chinese medicine. I would first and foremost like to thank the many translators, students, and teachers of Chinese medicine in both the United States and China who agreed to participate in this research, letting me observe their work and their classes, sitting through extensive interview sessions, and reading various drafts of this text. This book truly would not exist without you.

As I argue translation in Chinese medicine to be an intersubjective product of multiple past and present conversations, the present work also stands as a coconstructed conversation with many scholars in anthropology, sociology, history, and linguistics, as well as practitioners of Chinese medicine. I would thus like to offer my deepest gratitude to many of my UCLA colleagues and mentors, including especially Linda Garro, Ka-Kit Hui, Elinor Ochs, Hongyin Tao, and Yunxiang Yan, all of whom have spent countless hours helping me weave multiple and disparate theoretical strands into a unique synthesis of ideas. At UCLA, I would also like to thank Niko Besnier, Carole Browner, Alessandro Duranti, Marian Katz, Michael Heim, John Heritage, Douglas Hollan, and Paul Kroskrity. In the field of clinical Chinese medicine, I would like to thank, in particular, Dan Bensky, Eric Brand, Bob Damone, Andrew Ellis, Robert Felt, Martha Fielding, Stacy Gomes, Marnae Ergil, Bob Flaws, Shelley Ochs, Jason Robertson, Z'ev Rosenberg, Nigel Wiseman, and Honora Lee Wolfe for supporting this project in so many ways from conception to completion. In the interdisciplinary world of academic Chinese medicine, which often overlaps with both anthropology and clinical practice, I thank Linda Barnes, Mitra Emad, Judith Farquhar, Charlotte Furth, Hannah Flesch, Marta Hanson, Elisabeth Hsu, Evelyn Ho, Li Zhaoguo, Vivienne Lo, Eric Karchmer, Volker Scheid, Pierce Salgeuro, Soyoung Suh, Sabine Wilms, Yuan Bing, Mei Zhan, and Zhu Jianping. I have received such immense guidance, support, and encouragement from each of you, and many of you have provided invaluable feedback at various stages in this work. I would also like to wholeheartedly thank my editor at Berghahn Books for being especially patient and painstaking throughout the process of developing this book.

Throughout the researching and writing of this book, my friends and family have provided so much of the heart that has made it possible for me to persevere. In particular, I would like to thank Erin Berkowitz, Jeffrey Boynton, Heidi Christensen, Robin Clark, Michael Divine, Eti Domb, Sarah Megan Heller, Liu Li, Violet McKeon, Pier Paulo, Seamus Smith, Katie Winters, and Amy Wong. My greatest debt of gratitude is perhaps to my parents and stepparents. Blythe Egan, Steven Pritzker, Mary Hawkins, and Craig Tannahill: thank you from the bottom of my heart. I would finally like to thank my beautiful and wildly intelligent daughter, Nadya Rose, for simply being herself and reminding me in so many ways to maintain a balanced approach in both work and play.

This research was funded by a number of organizations at different stages of the work, including the Jacob K. Javits Graduate Research Fellowship (U.S. Department of Education), UCLA Graduate Division, and the Wenner-Gren Foundation for Anthropological Research.

Copyrights

Note on the Text

Transcription Conventions

Adapted from G. Jefferson, 1984

Throughout this text, the following transcription conventions are used:
The length of pauses are indicated in parentheses, with (.) indicating minute pauses.
Italicized words indicate accentuated speech.
Actions are indicated in ((double parentheses)).
Overlapped speech is marked by [brackets]
Drawn out words include a double colon (e.g., me::dicine)
The degree sign ° indicates that the talk following it is quiet or soft.
Up and down arrow marks indicate sharper rises or falls in pitch.
Capitalized text indicates SHOUTED or increased volume speech.
A question mark (?) indicates rising pitch or intonation.
A period (.) indicates falling pitch or intonation.
An equal sign (=) indicates the break and subsequent continuation of a single utterance.
A comma (,) indicates a temporary rise or fall in intonation.

Introduction

In Search of Resonance

A good translator … is also a good listener.
—Stéphanie Roesler, "Yves Bonnefoy's Metaphors on Translation"

I am sitting in a classroom along with about fifteen students who have just begun their four-year program at a school of Oriental Medicine in Southern California. At the end of this program, the students will take both state and national licensing exams to become practitioners of acupuncture and herbal medicine, along with—as they see fit to incorporate—Chinese medical massage, nutrition, and exercise. The teacher, a young non-Chinese speaking Caucasian man who himself has been licensed for about five years, launches into an extensive explanation of why translators who use the term "meridian" to translate the Chinese term 经络 *jingluo* are translating inaccurately. "The reason I don't like the word meridian is because it refers to—it's a name given by the French to like lay lines on the earth." He goes on to describe the origin of this mistranslation to the twentieth-century French translator Georges Soulié de Morant, differentiating the Chinese medical idea of "acupuncture channel" (his preferred translation) from "meridian" by saying, "I don't like to think of channels as imaginary lines. Meridians are man-made—we define what those are. To me, the channel is something that's there, that we use." This is followed by a lengthy digression into the history of Chinese medical transmission to Europe, through Soulié de Morant. A non-Chinese speaking student then asks what the Chinese term is, and the teacher responds by bringing in yet another Chinese term, 脉 *mai,* and the alternative translation, "vessel." The precise distinctions among *jingluo, mai,* channels (or meridians), and vessels are left unsettled.

A few months later, I sit comfortably on the couch with a cup of tea in the home office of a prominent translator of classical Chinese medicine, someone who has also taught in several U.S. schools of Oriental medicine. I have known her for several years, and the atmosphere is friendly and relaxed. I have a list of preestablished interview questions at hand, which I reach for from time to time throughout our conversation. As we address each of the questions, including queries into how she became interested in Chinese medicine, her experience with translation, and her perspectives on the available English-language literature, the conversation wanders and new questions arise. There is a great deal of laughter and many trips to a set of nearby bookshelves.

Together poring over both English-language and Chinese texts, we look at the ways in which Chinese authors and Western translators have approached the many thorny issues related to terminology selection, the ambiguity of ancient Chinese, and the need to distinguish Chinese medical terms from those of biomedicine. She comments on the ways in which each and every decision in her work translating ancient texts leads her back along a complex journey through the literature. Many Chinese authors throughout the ages, she reminds me, have produced commentaries on original texts. Such commentaries, which are inevitably based on the particular authors' own practice or scholarship, are critical resources for this translator, who tends to work on esoteric, ancient Chinese originals that are presented in sparse, ambiguous language. When two commentators differ in their explanations of an original text, something that happens often, she must weigh those differences and conduct even more research into still other texts before deciding how to frame her translation. Translating one sentence can take an entire week or more and may also involve several phone calls and e-mails to scholars she knows who specialize in the Chinese medical literature from different time periods.

From even these brief ethnographic scenes, it becomes clear that in the work of translating, and the work of teaching or learning Chinese medicine, the practicalities and contingencies of translation refuse to disappear. The ideal of seamless transfer of meaning, from one linguistic and cultural context to another, is illusive. There are hiccups, gaps, and critical junctures where the work of translating even one word can lead down a tortuous rabbit hole of history, shifting perspectives, and multiple interpretations. This book documents some of these trajectories, examining the seemingly endless series of conversations and practices that, somehow, despite all of the trials and tribulations, bring Chinese medicine to life in English so that it can be studied, learned, and practiced by Westerners who speak little to no Chinese.

This book is not a guidebook on translating Chinese medicine—far from it. Nor is it an attempt to describe objectively the process of translating Chinese medicine, the ways in which meaning is constructed through translation. Instead, it is an ethnographic portrayal of the variable ways in which translation, from Chinese to English (and sometimes back), is *enacted* in Chinese medicine. I use the term *enact* in the sense described by Mol, when she writes about the enactment of disease, through language, through practice, and also through objects (2002: 33). For translation to be enacted in Chinese medicine, then, there is quite obviously language—in books, but also in phone calls between translators who need to consult each other, in the classroom among students as they study together in groups, in the clinic as practitioners and patients talk, as well as in the varying selection of language used to designate Chinese medicine in the West (e.g., "Oriental medicine," "Traditional Chinese Medicine (TCM)," or "East Asian Medicine").[1] Here, there is not even just spoken or written language. There is gesture, intonation, and insinuated meaning. There is also practice: practices of inscribing or writing, but also practices of diagnosing, treating, acting upon real bodies in time, intervening in the course of illness, searching for meanings that resonate with felt realities. There are objects too. One thinks immediately, again, of books, and more books—original texts, commentaries, compiled translations, pamphlets, student notebooks, clinical handbooks, dictionaries (so many dictionaries: specialized medical dictionaries, etymological dictionaries, reverse dictionaries, historical dictionaries, electronic dictionaries—the list could go on). But there are also acupuncture needles and medicinal products—herbs, minerals, prepared formulas in capsules, teas, pills—along with massage tables, heat lamps, white coats, and moxa sticks. From the "praxiographic" view advocated by Mol (2002), none of these can be isolated from the enactment of translation in Chinese medicine.

With all of this to consider, one might also say that what I am attempting to demonstrate is the ways in which Chinese medicine in all of its facets is itself enacted through translation. From this vantage point, one might then say that I am looking at how acupuncture, herbal medicine, Chinese nutrition, and massage—how all of these things become real, are brought to bear in the context of very real clinical encounters—through the set of practices, the objects, and the conversations that make up translation in this vast field. This is a far-reaching goal. The scale of such an endeavor is probably beyond the scope of any one book. I will therefore stick with describing the enactment of translation itself rather than attempting to cover the enactment of Chinese medicine more broadly, doing my best to keep in mind that the enactment of anything in Chinese medicine necessarily entails all of these conversations, these practices, these objects.

To trace the enactment of translation in Chinese medicine, I conducted an ethnographic study that included interviews with translators, publishers, and scholars involved in the production of English-language educational material in the field of Chinese medicine in both China and the United States. Taking me from the headquarters of the World Federation of Chinese Medicine Societies (WFCMS) in Beijing to People's Medical Health Publishers (also in Beijing), to the academic offices of professors, scholars, and practitioners throughout China, the work in China consisted of a great deal of talking, reading, and searching through dictionaries. It was likewise in the United States, where I visited the three major publishers of English-language Chinese medical texts, companies that, staffed with in-house translators and authors and equipped with their own translation policies, produce most of the texts required by students to pass state and national boards in the United States. I interviewed many independent translators as well. At times, these interviews felt like tiny portholes into a vast ocean of translation work being conducted by more individuals than I could ever hope to convince to sit down and talk to me. Most of the more productive and well-known translators did eventually capitulate to my requests, however. Several refused; whether this was due to their busy schedules or due to my positioning in the field (see below), I will never necessarily know. Others I missed simply due to the sheer volume of scholars working in the field. I was, however, able to gather material from a good number of key translators and authors. Over the course the research in both the United States and China, I further attended several conferences and professional meetings pertaining to the translation of Chinese medicine, including several translation and terminology debates and workshops.

For an ethnographer, conducting interviews, attending conferences, and examining books is never enough. To ground the study in the everyday worlds of people using the texts created at my other fieldsites, I also conducted twenty-four months of ethnography in a Southern California school of Chinese medicine. This school, like many of the other twenty or so Acupuncture and Oriental Medicine (AOM) schools in California, consists of a four-year master's program that includes about three thousand hours of instruction in Chinese medical theory, biomedicine, acupuncture, herbal medicine, massage, and movement therapy. To sit for both the national and state board licensing exams, students must also participate in an eight-hundred-hour internship in a community clinic, usually associated with the school. Demographics at the site where the research was collected are similar to the general trend for California schools: about 70 percent of the students are Caucasian, 20 percent Asian, and 10 percent are of African American, Hispanic, or of Persian descent. About 60 percent of faculty are native English speakers, mostly Caucasian. The other 40 percent of faculty are Asian, mostly trained in Chinese and Taiwanese institutions, but also including Vietnamese, Korean, and Japanese trained practitioners. The majority of students are women (about 70 percent), and the age of students ranges from twenty to sixty, with an average age of thirty-two. About half of students have worked in the healthcare industry prior to starting school, and about the same amount have begun their studies as a direct result of having a positive personal experience with acupuncture. Most students enter the program with a bachelor's degree and pursue full-time study throughout their four years.

While at the school, I attended and video-recorded the entire first year of Chinese medical theory courses as well as second-, third-, and fourth-year classes in case management, needling, massage, tai chi (*taiji*), and Chinese medical language. During these classes, I also took extensive field notes. In addition to collecting classroom data, I conducted audio-recorded, open-ended interviews with several of the students and teachers who attended classes I recorded. I also spent a great deal of time at the school getting to know the students: I hung out in the break room, I accompanied them to lunch, and I had long conversations with them about their classes and texts. I pored through their textbooks and notes and became good friends with many of them. After the initial eighteen months of research was complete, I maintained ongoing relationships with several study participants and continued doing interviews and visiting with them at school over the course of their entire four-year program.

It is important to note here that I am a graduate of a similar California program and a longtime participant in and observer of language and translation debates in Chinese medicine, an arena in which many of my interviewees, both Chinese and Euro-American, are highly active. Further, my positioning as a licensed practitioner of acupuncture and Chinese medicine in California, a researcher at UCLA David Geffen School of Medicine's Center for East-West Medicine, and a teacher of Chinese language in a major California school of Chinese medicine, makes this project, in many ways, a "native ethnography." For these reasons, the current book is not necessarily objective in the sense that it studies a distinct other. At times "other," at times "self," the participants in this study have consistently forced me to consider my own shifting position(s) regarding translation in Chinese medicine, both as an anthropologist (because I am also that) *and* a practitioner in twenty-first-century U.S. practice. In this sense, a certain tension underlies much of the work. As Abu-Lughod puts it, "Because of their split selves, feminist and halfie anthropologists travel uneasily between speaking 'for' and speaking 'from'" (Abu-Lughod 1991: 143). For me, the uneasiness has come from wanting to pay extra care toward listening compassionately to every translator, every teacher, and every student, even when they are radically opposed. It has meant distancing myself from the temptation to draw premature conclusions based on convincing arguments. It has also meant nurturing my own "multiplex subjectivity" (Rosaldo 1989: 168–195, as cited in Narayan 1993: 676) in such a way as to create a product that seeks not only to describe the situation but also to contribute to the healing of what I see as some serious disparities in a highly charged and ethically situated field. Although it has often generated a great deal of discomfort for myself, and sometimes for participants (especially those expecting me to adhere to their positions, or who saw my previous work in the field as indexical of a view that contradicted their own), the tension of being a full participant as well as an engaged observer has proven to be the glue that has held this whole project together and has hopefully generated a useful contribution not only to the field of anthropology, but also to Chinese medicine.

Tracing Webs of Translation

Throughout all of this—the interviews, the travels, the readings, the observations—I often felt as though I were grasping at the ineffable, a moving target. The metaphors that are widely available for thinking about translation, for example, translation as an act of "smuggling" or otherwise carrying across, as an imperfect rendition, a deceitful performance, a transformation, were often inadequate on their own for thinking through the enactment of translation in Chinese medicine. Such images of betrayal, confusion, imitation, and treason are central to any discussion of translation and are apparent especially in positivist discourses in which the task of the translator hinges upon a Platonic differentiation of truth and form. In this scenario, the translator's burden is understood to be the expression of an essential truth in another form, the carrying of meaning across a divide that exists between a single "source language" toward a single "target language" (Van Wyke 2010). These metaphors are, of course, widely drawn upon in talk about translation in Chinese medicine. Here, translation is envisaged as an ethical act of representation in which one degrades the original message by polluting it with traces of the self. Translation in this view is violent, disruptive, and perfunctory.

Many participants in this study view translation in such terms, and I will talk extensively about their views in this book. But over the course of this research, I also witnessed another kind of enactment of translation, something more intimate, ongoing, dialogic, and emergent. Here, I witnessed translation unfold as a series of urgent, passionate, and life-changing conversations. These conversations are not rigid transactions or simple transfers of inert material, nor are they limited to definite junctures in time and space. The interlocutors include ancient authors and commentators, as well as contemporary translators, interpreters, and authors. But even, and perhaps especially, beyond the textually based translation of Chinese medicine, the ongoing event of translation continues as teachers, students, and patients participate actively in taking up and retranslating the work of experts.

These ongoing translation activities, springing forth from deeply felt desires to access another world, another language, another practice, and another culture, are not just searches for "the right words." In one crucial sense, they are a search for an authentic understanding of, and method for rerendering, the linguistic practice of Chinese medicine as it evolved in China and beyond. The many engagements and conversations with texts, teachers, patients, friends, and colleagues are also, however, a search for the self, a search for wholeness, spirituality, for authentic, effective practice, and for a language that addresses the real needs of patients. In the process of conducting the research, as a result of a distinctive person-centered ethnographic approach (Hollan 2001, 2005; Levy and Hollan 1998), I thus developed close relationships with several students, who are featured regularly throughout the book. Over the course of the next seven chapters, then, you will repeatedly see excerpts from interviews and classroom segments involving Julia, Treavor, Sarah, Tanya, and Oren.[2] Each of these students became involved with Chinese medicine for various personal reasons, but all of them were in some way inspired by the desire for a career promising to be spiritually fulfilling and offering the opportunity to participate in an alternative paradigm of and the body. For these students, conversations about translation are also often a search for hope, for relationship, for a better model with which to think about the body, to heal illness, and to transform a rapidly demoralizing American healthcare system. Throughout all of this, no part of the self is left untouched. Cryptic words are digested, medicines are consumed, layers of the mind and body are dissected, and old wounds are healed.

For this reason, I began to identify more with dialogic metaphors and ways of thinking through translation, finding myself drawn to images of breath, rhythm, and relationship in translation. The French contemporary poet and translator Yves Bonnefoy, for example, highlights the importance of intense *listening* before beginning the *intimate conversation* that is translation (Roesler 2010). Bonnefoy's metaphors are thus full of encounters and close interactions in which the author is a friend, neighbor, and fellow traveler (Roesler 2010: 217). Walking together along the path of speech, the two writers engage in a sensual exchange in which the rhythm of the original author's core self can be, through a close, embodied listening, "transmitted from the poet's body to the translator's" (Roesler 2010: 224). This transfer unfolds through feeding on or breathing in the sound, texture, and meaning of the original, literally ingesting the words into oneself. Bonnefoy further speaks of developing a new self-understanding through this process and ultimately expressing the rhythm of the new self in the final translation. For Bonnefoy, respect is located in the relationship one forms with the original author, and authentic translation unfolds as a merging of voices involved in a dialogic encounter. The key, for him, is learning to listen.

Other translators talk about their work in similar terms. Edith Grossman, for example, writes about listening, saying that "[i]n the process of translating, we endeavor to hear the first version of the work as profoundly and completely as possible, struggling to discover the linguistic charge, the structural rhythms, the subtle implications, the complexities of meaning and suggestion in vocabulary and phrasing, and the ambient, cultural inferences and conclusions these tonalities allow us to extrapolate" (2010: 8–9). Like Bonnefoy, Grossman is here talking about a deeply dialogic and embodied encounter. "This is a kind of reading as deep as any encounter with a literary text can be," she continues (2010: 8–9). Encounters with language in Chinese medicine, I noticed over the course of this study, are equally deep and equally personal.

Resonance is therefore another metaphor that I draw upon for understanding translation. Resonance, or 感应 *ganying*, is often described in Chinese medicine as the connection between practitioner and patient, the "permeability between persons and things" (Zhuo 2007: 383) that allows for deep recognition and deep healing. In Chinese philosophy more generally, resonance describes the architecture of the universe as a series of "endless chains of correspondences between different parts" (Le Blanc 1995: 73). To know these chains is to *feel* them, with the first character in the term, *gan*, referring to affect, and the second, *ying*, designating a reaction or response. This type of knowing is inherently transformative, for all participants. It is a felt engagement that emerges through relationship, an embodied equivalence that is not dependent on words per se but that is disclosed in language. Throughout this book, I will therefore speak repeatedly of the search for resonance on the part of translators, teachers, students, and interns. I see this search for connection or relationship with the language of Chinese medicine as the heart of many aspects of translation.

The conversations that surround, implicate, and even generate translation in Chinese medicine are not "just personal," however, nor could they be. Complex politics and relations of power play an enormous role in shaping the ways in which such conversations unfold in the everyday lives of participants. If in the more dialogic metaphors of translation described above, translation begins with a deep listening to original author(s), the task of contemporary translators and interpreters of Chinese medicine is greatly challenged by the need to learn *how* to listen in a field of multiple voices resounding interdiscursively through thousands of years of texts, politics, and practice. Many of these voices are saying vastly different things about tradition, history, authenticity, and the self. Within this cacophony, there are claims that certain voices want to drown out the sounds and rhythms of the thousands of Chinese authors who have developed the tradition over time (see, for example, Emad 2006 or Scheid 2007). This is where the imaging of translation in Chinese medicine takes on a distinctly ethical tone, and metaphors of smuggling or transforming come back to the fore, raising questions about who is authorized to participate, how much Chinese one needs to speak to participate, and what role self-knowledge or clinical experience plays in the process. Debates are lively. And within all of the intimate engagements that unfold in these interactive spaces, long-lasting relationships and institutions are formed. Here, I found myself drawn to the metaphor of translation as landscape, an image that acknowledges the instability of translations as they are produced and received in various environments (Kershaw and Saldanha 2013).

Living Translation

The disparate nature of this process, this enactment, demanded a dynamic theory of translation that could, if not capture, then at least attend to all of these different phases or aspects of translation as it is enacted in Chinese medicine—the exchanges between students and teachers, the experience of translators as well as consumers of translation, and the sociocultural power dynamics involved with translating. In search of such a comprehensive theory, I combed through studies of translation in anthropology, sociology, sociolinguistics, and translation studies. The result of my search—less a theory and more like a framework for thinking about translation in Chinese medicine—is what I call "living translation." Specifically, living translation points to the way translation in Chinese medicine is enacted through inscription, interaction, embodied experience, and practice into multiple spoken and written forms that challenge binary notions of power and difference.

Living translation is crafted, in part, after MacIntyre's (2007 [1981]) notion of "living tradition," especially as developed by Scheid (2007). MacIntyre, who recognizes the dynamic nature of tradition, focuses on the involvement of diverse and often disagreeing participants in the creation of tradition. These "continuities of conflict" inspire a rethinking of the role of interaction, practice, and relationship in the building of "an historically extended, socially embodied argument" (MacIntyre 2007 [1981]: 222). Scheid, in an exploration of certain forms of practice in Chinese medicine, thus shows how narratives of tradition, over time and through ongoing interactions and transactions, are both continued and remade into "currents" that flow recognizably through time despite their constant renegotiation. Viewing translation through this lens reveals it as similarly ongoing, emerging in multiple acts of retranslation that position actors within a social world where participants have varying access to source texts and meanings are made and remade in open-ended and ongoing "living narratives" (Ochs and Capps 2001) that both continue and transform linguistic, personal, and social meanings.

The notion of interaction, or more specifically conversation, a concept I have already invoked repeatedly in this introduction, is a crucial component of this perspective. I envision conversation, following Hans-Georg Gadamer, as a process of "coming to an understanding," "a dialectic "event" that is disclosed in language (Gadamer 2004 [1975]: 443). "You understand a language," writes

Gadamer, "by living in it" (2004 [1975]: 386). All parties who are involved in this lived event, and here I include readers and interpreters as well as authors and translators, together embark on a journey where they "fall into" or "become involved in" conversation, often being led into an unknown realm through an engagement with one another (Gadamer 2004 [1975]: 385). This interpretive transformation often occurs across the "abyss of historical consciousness" (Gadamer 1981: 98) and incorporates a further transformation in self-understanding, which, being "always on-the-way" (1981: 103), is enhanced by the interaction. "Understanding is an adventure," Gadamer writes, "and, like any other adventure, is dangerous" (1981: 109–110).

This notion of conversation as adventure implies a generative and transformative merging of predispositions that recalls Bonnefoy's metaphors of intimate engagement and transformation in the process of translation. On translation, Gadamer thus similarly highlights the multiple relationships that unfold in the multiplex interaction. "Translation," Gadamer suggests, "is an extreme case that doubles the hermeneutical process … there is one conversation between the interpreter and the other, and a second between the interpreter and oneself" (Gadamer 2004 [1975]: 387). Although Gadamer's theories have been criticized for being idealistic and unable to attend to the discrepancies in power in translative encounters (Lianeri 2002), it is a useful metaphor for understanding living translation as a series of involved conversations. Complemented by Bonnefoy's images of intimacy, sensuality, and the difficulty of true listening, Gadamer's notion of conversation can also serve as a foundation for understanding the uneven and very personal nature of many of the dialogues that together comprise the living translation of Chinese medicine.

As such, living translation incorporates moments of authoring, experiences with reading, encounters with teachers, colleagues, friends, and patients. It also includes private moments of embodied learning and intercorpreal moments of engaging with bodies in practice. Living translation weaves together morally situated desires for authenticity with culturally grounded notions of healing in everyday practices of writing and teaching about Chinese medicine. It is about learning specific words, but also about ways of speaking, ways of interacting, and ways of being. In this sense, living translation can be conceived as ongoing, emerging in multiple acts of retranslation that position actors within a social world where participants have varying access to source texts and meanings are made and remade in narratives that both continue and transform linguistic, personal, and social meanings. At the same time, living translation acknowledges the mediating role of various moral frameworks, objects (including texts), historical and institutional practices, as well as ideologies of language and translation that inform and regulate the moments where inscriptions, interactions, embodied experiences, and practice enact the translation of Chinese medicine.

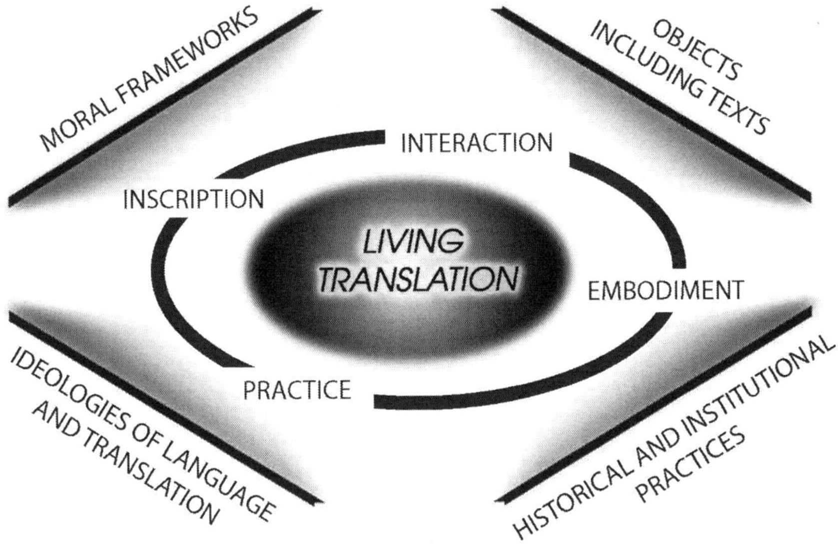

These multiple processes are constantly in motion, interpenetrating one another with shifting perspectives and continuously generating multiple "results." Within such a framework, translation can be and often is multiple things: a smuggling, an act of violence, a deep listening, and a shifting landscape.

To be clear, living translation is a collage of sorts, an attempt to draw together multiple disciplinary views on translation in a framework for understanding the process of translation in Chinese medicine as I was witnessing it in my research. From translation studies, it draws upon the work of scholars who highlight the ethical engagement of translators and interpreters as they negotiate the power and responsibility inherent in the bridging of cultural and linguistic divides (Asad 1986; Bermann and Wood 2005; Friedrich 1992 [1965]; Nietzsche 1992 [1882]; Schliermacher 1992 [1813]; Tymoczko and Gentzler 2002; Venuti 2000, 2005). Here, the notions of appropriation and colonization of source material through translation provide a lens through which to view some of the transformations that take place in the translation of Chinese medicine. But living translation also incorporates work in translation studies that emphasizes the dialogic nature of translation (Wadensjö 1998), the chain of correspondence through which the "idiosomatic force" of translation emerges through both production and reception of specific works (Robinson 1991). Living translation as well draws upon studies that emphasize a rethinking of translation through the metaphor of the landscape (Kershaw and Saldanha 2013), a notion that is heavily influenced by the work of sociocultural anthropologists such as Appadurai and Bhabha (see Appadurai 1996; Bhabha 1994). These perspectives invite the view of translation in Chinese medicine as taking place in multiple concurrent practices: writing, reading, feeling, talking, and practicing.

Living translation in Chinese medicine is further theoretically grounded in the linguist and literary scholar Roman Jakobson's distinctions among "intralingual," "interlingual," and "intersemiotic" translation (1966 [1959]: 233). Whereas interlingual translation is the term Jakobson uses to define what is commonly understood as "translation proper" or "an interpretation of verbal signs by means of some other language" (1966 [1959]: 233), *intra*lingual translation refers to "an interpretation of verbal signs by other signs of the same language" (1966 [1959]: 233). In intralingual translation, then, concepts are translated vis-à-vis a "circumlocution" that functions to define or describe their meaning. Intersemiotic translation, on the other hand, is "interpretation of verbal signs by means of signs of nonverbal sign systems" (1966 [1959]: 233). Living translation sits at the intersection of all of these forms of translation, incorporating the interlingual shifts between Chinese and English as well as the multiple interpretive moments where Chinese terms are interpreted through extended intralingual explanations and intersemiotic demonstrations of meaning in English.

Work in science studies, history, and Chinese studies also inform the development of living translation. Larissa Heinrich, for example, looks at the translation of the Western anatomical body in eighteenth-century China, focusing especially on the translation of images and the ways in which such images functioned to challenge and transform fundamental categories such as the self, the notion of evidence, and the boundaries of the human body in China (Heinrich 2008). In this work, Heinrich notes the special role of translations enacted through collaboration between specific Westerners and Chinese authors, physicians, and artists, with translations emerging as "a kind of unmediated, or less mediated, translated text: they were the direct product of a cross-cultural conversation and as such represented a cooperative attempt to arrive at a new, hybrid visual idiom" (Heinrich 2008: 43). In another historical study, Scott Montgomery traces the translation of scientific concepts throughout history, focusing especially on the translation of astronomy from Greek to Roman to Arabic to Japanese. "Translation," he writes, "is not a word that describes any single activity" (Montgomery 2000: 3). Montgomery thus reveals translation as an ongoing "process of communication" (2000: 4) involving disparate sets of imagined originals and equally variable renditions created by multiple authors with differing levels of skill in both the languages they write in and the practices they write about. This hive of activity results in an ever-expanding "array of works" (Montgomery 2000: 286) within which it is apparent that each act of translation is embedded in a series of ongoing social processes much more complex than the simple source-target model allows. In this perspective, there is seldom a pure source and a clear target. Instead of one source and one target, one original and one translation, the socially situated practice of transmission reveals that translation in real sociocultural circumstances, especially over time, often makes the identification of a single, true source extremely complex. From this perspective, at each level of translation there exist multiple personal, cultural, and institutional "voices" that infuse the concepts with many layers of meaning that cannot be designated as either source or target, but that are themselves produced in the conversation. In Chinese medicine, the multiplicity of texts and interpretations of texts demands such a view.

In many ways, the "big picture" view invites an attendance to what Lydia Liu, another major influence on living translation, refers to as "translingual practice":

> Broadly defined, the study of translingual practice examines the process by which new words, meanings, discourses, and modes of representation arise, circulate, and acquire legitimacy within the host language due to, or in spite of, the latter's contact/collision with the guest language. Meanings, therefore, are not so much "transformed" when concepts pass from the guest language to the host language as invented within the local environment of the latter (Liu 1995: 26).

Like Montgomery, Liu brings attention to multiple social encounters that influence meaning when it comes to transmitting language. Especially when it involves an ongoing practice, Liu emphasizes, "One must account for the complexities of the trajectory of a discourse" (Liu 1995: 66). For Liu, the prioritization of the social trajectory of translations precludes arguments over commensurability, calling the researcher's attention away from what is not accomplished in translation to what *is*. This draws the ethnographer of translation in Chinese medicine to look at how translation is being enacted in real situations of writing, learning, speaking, and practicing, rather than focusing on how it should be done or could otherwise have been done if more rigorous linguistic principles had been applied. The shift here is from language to the people using the language.

Several anthropologists and other social scientists have likewise underscored the role of people in the translation of any cultural practice, emphasizing human relationships, power, understanding, and interaction in the translation process (Abel 2005; Appiah 2000 [1993]; Aravamudan 2006; Clifford 1997; Hanks 2010; Hart 1999; Herzfield 2003; Rubel and Rosman 2003; Sagli 2010; Schieffelin 2007, 2008; Silverstein 2003; Strauss 2005; Tambiah 1990; Tymoczko and Gentzler 2002; Zhan 2009). For example, Hanks (2010) offers a rich historical analysis of the use of translation in the Spanish conquest of the Yucatan, demonstrating how exploited populations came to use the invented language of *Maya reducido,* with its foundation in Christian ideology, to develop identities and texts that were eventually used to challenge colonizers. "In the age of the cross," he writes, "words designed to convert had themselves been converted" (2010: 371). From this vantage point, power is not as simple as a single dominant group exerting influence over a single subjugated group through violent acts of translation. Bambi Schieffelin (2007, 2008) focuses on the role of translation in the Christianization of the Bosavi and shows in particular how deeply embedded epistemologies of the self, language, and culture can be accessed through a focus on translation activities. With this work, she further demonstrates the role of translation in shifting culturally embedded ways of being-in-the world, all the while highlighting the role of individual actors—translators, interpreters, audience members—in facilitating this process. The work of Hanks and Schieffelin both value a close ethnographic examination of the ways in which translated words, and translated texts, are received among individuals in complex life circumstances. In the present study, this invites a closer look at the ways in which particular students and practitioners in the West engage with translations in both the study and practice of Chinese medicine.

Finally, several anthropologists have contributed specifically to the study of translation in Chinese medicine. Mitra Emad, for example, discusses the body as a site for the cultural translation of Chinese medicine in the West, arguing that "[w]hile acupuncture clearly provides pain relief, it also offers an opportunity to explore [one's] body ... pointing to a very different map of the body than most of us carry with us on a daily basis" (1998: 154). The body itself is thus translated through acupuncture, and the role of acupuncturists in providing this opportunity for American patients positions them as "cultural translators of an alternative medical worldview" (Emad 1998: 44). Mei Zhan further demonstrates the translocal production of Chinese medicine in the everyday "encounters and entanglements" of involved participants (2009: 12), including practitioners, teachers, politicians, patients, and students in both China and the United States. Based on research in Shanghai and San Francisco, Zhan's work examines the process of cultural translation as it unfolds in various historical, social, and political circumstances. Zhan thus approaches Chinese medicine as a socially emergent network, espousing a sociocultural view that looks at interactions over time as constitutive of practice. In focusing on socialities, Zhan asks her readers to understand the "worlding" of Chinese medicine as an ongoing spaciotemporal process involving multiple relationships and "zones of encounter" negotiated "in action" (2009: 12). Both Emad's incorporation of the body in the translation of Chinese medicine, as well as Zhan's perspective on translation in Chinese medicine as emergent in multiple social networks provide a strong foundation for the current discussion of living translation in Chinese medicine.

Building on Emad and Zhan's work, as well as the emerging multidisciplinary understanding of translation as dialogic, personal process, the current study focuses specifically on language, closely examining the everyday interactions that constitute the linguistic, as opposed to cultural, Chinese-English translation of Chinese medicine. When I speak of language, here, I am referring not only to individual words and terms, although that certainly is a large part of it, but also to indexically grounded language as both a social process as well as "as a mode of experiencing the world in itself" (Ochs 2010: 6). In this sense, I look at the experiences of authors engaging with multiple source texts and multiple target audiences in their efforts to create the language in which Chinese medicine is experienced by students in the United States. I also look at the collaborative nature of translation in the classroom and clinical context, including the embodied experience of students as well as patients, all as part of the entire intertextual and intersubjective project of searching for ways of thinking about, speaking about, and finding resonance with Chinese medicine in English. Living translation thus draws from many disciplines, both theoretically and methodologically. Within each chapter, much of this literature—spanning linguistic anthropology, medical and psychological anthropology, sociolinguistics, history, and translation studies—is drawn upon to elucidate the data. Living translation, as depicted above, is maintained throughout the text as the overall taxonomy of translation in Chinese medicine. The book is thus organized according to different phases of living translation, but each chapter contains seeds of the process of the whole. Likewise, as a product, the current volume is also in many ways a part of the living translation process, as especially in the case of translation, one can never separate the work of explanation through ethnography from the translation process itself (Anelo 2005; Rubel and Rosman 2003).

Writing Trajectory

Following this introduction, chapters 1 and 2 describe the outer ring in the diagram above: the historical and institutional practices, the moral frameworks, the objects, and the ideologies of language and translation in Chinese medicine. Chapter 1 is organized around two ethnographic vignettes collected at the U.S. school of Chinese medicine where this research was carried out, and through the lens of these vignettes situates contemporary Chinese medical practice in the transnational framework of twentieth-century healthcare practices, including the introduction of biomedicine in China and the emerging importance of complementary and alternative (CAM) therapies in the United States. This includes a discussion of the historical and institutional frameworks in the development of the multiple forms of Chinese medicine in both the United States and China, as well as both the moral landscape and material goods that shape this development and mediate the enactment of Chinese-English translation.

In chapter 2, "Ideas about Words, and Words about Ideas," I focus specifically on ideologies of language and translation in Chinese medicine, drawing upon interview data from students and teachers of Chinese medicine in the United States as well as public statements made by authors, translators, and consumers participating in the international translation and terminology debates in Chinese medicine. By "ideologies of language and translation," I am referring specifically to ideas about what people in the field of Chinese medicine think language and translation are and how they understand what language and translation do or should do (see Kroskrity 2004; Silverstein 1979). As with the moral landscape, the ideological landscape is portrayed in this chapter as a set of available ideas that participants variably draw upon in their quest to learn, teach, translate, and practice Chinese medicine in English.

Chapter 3, "Living Inscription in Chinese Medicine," focuses on specific translators and translations, drawing upon both interview and textual data to examine the socially, politically, culturally, personally, and morally situated search for valid kinds of equivalence. Here, I demonstrate that textuality in Chinese medicine is a richly interdiscursive and lively process, a mode of social action that is ongoing as authors create texts as conversations with past, present, and future practice (Hanks 1989). The social act of translation in Chinese medicine thus requires authors to position themselves and their work vis-à-vis multiple, shifting communities of practice, past, present, and future. All of these different laminations articulate with the daily practice and personal perspectives of translators as they create new work, respond to others' work, and engage in conversations with students about their work. It is this complexity that makes translation in Chinese medicine, already at the level of the text, a living process involving multiple, ongoing searches for resonance and meaning.

Chapter 4, "Interaction in the Living Translation of Chinese Medicine," focuses on daily interactive practices that unfold in the classroom as teachers and students engage in "translation talk" in response to the multiple translations they are confronted with in their texts. Here, I show how students learn, from the beginning of their program, to "do" translation as a core part of their developing practice. I further show how teachers use variable "evidentiality strategies" (Aikhenvald 2004) for translation as a positioning tool to establish their authority to participate in the translation and interpretation of key terms and concepts. Finally, I show how specific translations emerge collaboratively through the interactive, mutually constitutive socialization of both students and teachers.

Chapter 5, "Embodied Experience in the Living Translation of Chinese Medicine," examines the ways in which everyday discourse about language in the school is not limited to talk. Students are also always actively searching for resonance in their embodied engagement with the terms and concepts of

Chinese medicine. They are guided in this endeavor by teachers and clinical instructors who encourage them to formulate their own vocabulary of the medicine based on their felt experience of feeling pulses, consuming herbs and other medicinal substances, and reflecting upon the self. Chapter 5 thus examines the ways in which both body and self become major mediums through which meaning is transmitted, and through which terms are translated, as students form a working relationship with the language of Chinese medicine.

Chapter 6, "Living Translation in and into Practice," shows how the living translation of Chinese medicine carries forth in the practice of acupuncture, medicinal prescription, and the pursuit of effective treatments that are resonant with patients' conditions. Here, I show how this translation emerges in everyday moments of communicative engagement where interns and practitioners translate Chinese terms for patients. Part performance, part patient socialization, translation in practice is an important opportunity for interns and practitioners to assert their authority, build rapport with patients, and start generating clinical results. In both translating for and upon patients, in this chapter I show how the living translation of Chinese medicine unfolds as a discursive, embodied, social, moral, political, and economic engagement that extends the texts, the classroom conversations, and the embodied learning examined in the previous chapters.

In the conclusion, "Learning to Listen," I revisit some of the metaphors of translation explored in this introduction, including especially the ways in which transformation variably figures into different notions of translation. Examining the linguistic, personal, and institutional transformations that issue forth from the process of living translation, I reexamine some of the culturally framed debates on translation in light of the current findings. I conclude with a brief discussion of living translation as a model with implications beyond Chinese medicine, specifically in the developing cross-disciplinary dialogue between multiple subfields of anthropology, translation studies, history, medicine, and Chinese studies.

Throughout all of the chapters, many different types of ethnographic data are drawn upon to raise questions, discuss theoretical frameworks, and elucidate multiple points of view. These data include my own observations, textual citations, quotes from participant interviews, and excerpts of classroom dialogue. In the representation of participants' speech gathered through interviews, I use a basic method of transcription that excludes most, though not all, nonverbal actions, including gestures, as well as vocal utterances such as repairs and pauses. For the sake of readability and space, such segments are selectively filtered such that the content of what is being described is clear. This is a compromise that I do not make in the representation of interactional excerpts from classroom dialogue that often involves more than one participant. In such cases, to demonstrate the interactional work that is being accomplished beyond language, I use a Jeffersonian transcription notation method that allows for the annotation of overlapping speech, pauses, ranges in pitch, gestures, and emphasis (Jefferson 1984). These transcription conventions are described in "Note on the Text: Transcription Conventions." Throughout the book, all Romanization for Chinese terms is in *hanyu pinyin.*

Notes

1. For a discussion of the politics of naming Chinese medicine in the United States, see Burke 2006.
2. All names are pseudonyms.

CHAPTER

1

The Real Chinese Medicine

At any point in its long evolution Chinese medicine has been characterized by a diversity that encompasses every aspect of its organization and practice, from theory and diagnosis to prognosis, therapeutics, and the social organization of healthcare.

—Volker Scheid, *Chinese Medicine in Contemporary China*

To attempt to define Chinese medicine is to become immediately embroiled in a complex web of sociocultural and historical circumstances stretching from the eighteenth century B.C. to the present, from Tibet to Mongolia to India to Europe to China and back again. Several renowned scholars have taken steps toward filling in pieces of this history, showing how the various practices and theories that comprise what is now understood as Chinese medicine have developed alongside vast political and social changes in China, and beyond, for several thousands of years (Furth 1999; Hinrichs and Barnes 2013; Kuriyama 1994; Scheid 2002, 2007; Sivin 1987; Taylor 2004; Unschuld 1985; Zhu 2002). Some of the same scholars have further demonstrated the inherent hybridity of Chinese medicine, where interaction with foreign ideas and people has played a critical role in shaping many past and current practices (Buell 1989; Scheid 2002). Especially in the last hundred years, Chinese medicine in both China and the United States has emerged as a continually shifting set of practices that is deeply intertwined with politics, culture, and the institutional practices of biomedicine.

It is from this vantage point that this chapter reviews the historical and institutional practices, the moral frameworks, and some of the material goods mediating the translation of Chinese medicine. The focus of this chapter, as in the book as a whole, is the United States. Because the historical, institutional, and moral frameworks permeating the translation of Chinese medicine in the United States are deeply intertwined with the development of Chinese medicine in China, the discussion also delves into some very broad Chinese history. I aim to show that in both China and the United States the stakes involved with authenticating medical practice have varied and have deeply influenced the way "the medicine" (as it is often called by practitioners and instructors in the United States) is enacted in both "original" and "translated" languages. In fact, one could argue that the shifting stakes are part and parcel of what makes it difficult to pinpoint what is original and what is translated, even within Chinese. A full discussion of this complexity is beyond the scope of this chapter. Rather than providing a comprehensive overview, then, by drawing upon ethnographic examples from my research, I dip in and out of this complex history to foreground some of the ways in which major historical, social, and cultural forces are coming together in the present, as the search for the "real" Chinese medicine in English-language translation unfolds as a deeply moral endeavor with far-reaching implications for translation and practice.

When I talk about the morality of this search, I am referring to ideas about what it means to be a "good" healer, what it means to be a good learner of Chinese medicine, and what it means to be a guardian of wisdom that is being transmitted across time, language, and culture. In this sense, I am referring to the questions that people ask about, as Charles Taylor puts it, "what kind of life is worth living ... or of what constitutes a rich, meaningful life" (1989: 14). Everyone participating in the practice, the teaching, or the translation of Chinese medicine in the United States has deeply personal answers to such questions. The answers are sometimes quite different and often are both fluid and subject to a great deal of ambivalence. The "moral landscape" of Chinese medicine, I suggest, is a heterogeneous arena in which "one observes a proliferation of types and figures of moral discourse ... both within collectivities and within individuals" (Rabinow 2008: 79). What I introduce in this chapter, and aim to show in the rest of this book, is that the project of authenticating Chinese medicine vis-à-vis these morally charged orientations toward the "goods" to which one aspires very much mediates the enactment of translation in both text and practice.

Looking toward the multiple and shifting moral "goods" of Chinese medicine quickly leads to an examination of the material goods, the objects involved in the enactment of translation, as well. "We usually think it is easy to distinguish ethical and aesthetic objects or issues," writes Taylor. "But when it is a matter of sentiments ... then the lines seem difficult to draw" (1989: 373–374). This chapter thus also includes some discussion of the "stuff" of Chinese medicine—the acupuncture needles, herbs and other medicinal substances, massage tables, crystals, blood vessels, muscles, and white doctor coats. Although books as objects of consumption also play an obvious role in the enactment of translation, and will come up repeatedly throughout this text, this chapter takes a broader view toward objects, avoiding the temptation to see such things simply "as things manipulated in practices" (Mol 2002: 4). Instead, following Mol, I do not isolate such objects from the enactment of translation in Chinese medicine, but view them to be as much a part of this enactment as words or books. A focus on acupuncture needles in particular facilitates this examination.

By describing the historical and institutional practices, the moral frameworks, and the objects of Chinese medicine in the United States, what I am presenting, together with the ideologies of language and translation described in the next chapter, can in some senses be seen as the stage upon which living translation progresses in Chinese medicine. This metaphor demonstrates the extent to which actors on this stage are positioned as translators who must bridge the tensions that pervade it. In the diagram that I offered in the introduction, these factors constitute the outer ring surrounding living translation as it is enacted in inscription, interaction, embodied experience, and practice. But again following Mol (2002), the stage metaphor runs dry, as it lends itself more to thinking about "context" as background, and action as "performance." If instead my goal is to focus on the enactment of translation in Chinese medicine, then it becomes more useful to think about this chapter as providing insight into the factors that mediate this enactment: history, morality, and materiality. To better understand what I mean by this, I begin this chapter with several ethnographic vignettes and return to discuss them only after several sections weaving together history, institutional practice, as well as both moral and material frameworks.

Ethnographic Orientations: Of Blood and Self-Discovery

To ground the following discussion of history, institutional practice, morality, and materiality that follows, I begin by describing two interactions, both of which took place during the first year of the four-year program in the school of Chinese medicine where I conducted my research. I share these particular interactive moments not because they are especially unique or notable. Instead, I offer them as commonplace exchanges in the everyday worlds of students learning Chinese medicine, everyday moments of questioning and learning what Chinese medicine *is* and how to speak about it. They are presented in this section without detailed analyses, which require more insight into the multiple historical, institutional, and moral frameworks mediating the enactment of translation in Chinese medicine. I therefore suggest possible specific analyses of the encounters only after presenting this complex terrain, not just as necessary "background" but as the very stuff—the environment—that creates the possibility for the interactions in the first place.

The first interaction I describe takes place in the first quarter class introducing the fundamentals of Oriental medicine to beginning students. The lecture has turned toward a discussion of blood and what is meant by the term "blood deficiency" in Chinese medicine. The Chinese term for blood, otherwise understood as the red fluid circulating throughout the body, is 血 *xue* (sometimes pronounced *xie*). In both Chinese medical contexts and biomedical contexts, the English translation is, simply, "blood." What is meant by this term differs, however, beyond the core feature of being red fluid circulating in the body. In biomedicine, *xue* circulates through arteries and veins and contains white and red blood cells, platelets, and proteins. In Chinese medicine, *xue* is also described in English translations as "the material foundation for the Mind" (Maciocia 2005: 60) or even as "being" itself (Kaptchuk 2000: 52). Described as "the soft, receptive part of the self" (Jarrett 1998: 305) or "the sense of authentic self," (Van Hoy 2010: 119), blood in translated Chinese medicine becomes both more central and more ambiguous. Given all of these various ways of understanding blood, the notion of "blood deficiency," a common diagnosis in Chinese medicine characterized by pale skin, weakness, palpitations, forgetfulness, fatigue, insomnia, or even a sense of "psychic vulnerability" or poor sense of self (Van Hoy 2010: 120), is difficult to grasp, especially for first-year students accustomed to biomedical categories such as anemia. Christine, a student with a background in biomedical nursing, thus asks her instructor, Carter, about the term "blood deficiency":

Chris: In blood deficiency? So what I'm thinking that you said was that the body's not producing enough (.) blood? So generally we have about 8, 5 liters of blood=excess liters of blood so actually less than that?

Carter: Ummm[mm]

Chris: [Volume] decreases?

Carter, their instructor, offers a lengthy response, building upon the possibility that a future patient will think that they are anemic when told that their diagnosis in Chinese medicine is "blood deficiency," or vice versa. After explaining that "we" could still diagnose them as being blood deficient even if their red blood cell count is fine, he explains "what we mean when we say blood":

Carter: You know, not necessarily—because um (2.0) people=more commonly the way that question is asked is you know, well do I have to go in and get—if I get the blood test, and it says I'm anemic, does that mean I'm blood deficient? And if it says I'm not anemic, does that mean I'm not blood deficient? And the answer's no. Um, there *is* some crossover, there's some correlation, ((interlinks fingers on hands)) but there's not a definitive (.) um one to one um (.) ah (.) connection that you can make with those so you know, we could have a patient who gets their blood work taken, right, and they check for anemia, and they're not—they're fine, right, their red blood cell count's fine. Um, but *we?* could still diagnose them as being blood deficient in this system, k? ((extends arms in parallel)) Um, so=and that's one of the

> instances where you have to think about, um (1.5) What do we mean when we say blood? Does it include what they're talking about? Is it also something else? And the answer is yes (.) um, we are talking about the Western version of blood, but it's also all these additional, you know, concepts associated with the blood in Chinese medicine, so (.) um the perspective is that we can detect, ah, blood deficiency=what you'd say in Western medicine is subclinical, all right=it's not going to appear on the laboratory test but our assumption is that left untreated, it ultimately *would,* right? We're just detecting it, um (.) before the test does.

In distinguishing between "blood" in Chinese and Western medicines, Carter here invokes the concept of "subclinical" to explain the reasons why a patient with blood deficiency would not necessarily be shown as having anemia on a lab test. He also builds a potential bridge by suggesting that blood deficiency is a kind of precursor to anemia, arguing that "if left untreated, it ultimately would [turn into anemia]." This leads into a longer, more extensive lecture about the ways in which "normal ranges" on biomedical laboratory tests are decided upon.

The second interaction I describe takes place in the second quarter "OM Diagnosis" class, where students learn the diagnostic techniques of Oriental medicine: looking at tongues, taking pulses, palpating bodies, and listening to patients' stories. In the following exchange, the students have just had a chance to practice feeling pulses for the first time. After working in pairs, the class has come back together to debrief. Julia talks about what she learned about herself during the exercise, how she relates her tendency to "go in too deep too fast" to her experience feeling her classmates' pulses. Her teacher, Barbara, responds:

Julia: I, um, in my massage therapy practice? the big (0.5) challenge that I've always had to have is to not go in too deep too fast. ((teacher laughs)) I just like [have]=

Barbara: [yeah]

Julia: =this tendency to really like—

Barbara: Surgical precision …

Julia: *And,* um, I don't— I *don't* mean to—I'm so unaware of it, it's unbelievable, and, and sometimes even when I'm consciously trying to be very—like people will tell me specifically to be soft, and I'll say, look, okay, be °sooo soft°, and people will still say, like, it was way too intense for me. And um, and so that's just something I'm kinda—and since, since I've started school here, it's (.) I—I've been able to articulate that? [I mean]=

Barbara: [yeah]

While Julia is talking, Barbara, a Caucasian woman who has been practicing for over ten years, nods, and laughs, expressing alignment by interjecting brief comments to show she understands what her student is saying and encouraging her self-reflection. Julia continues, explaining that she's only been able really to articulate this tendency in herself since she's been in the program. She further relates her experience with the pulse to this new understanding of herself:

Julia: You know, and—and with the pulses just now, I felt it very profoundly, like that when I would go on I just felt like that there was a *hole,* I just got sucked in, ((continuously draws hands toward body)) and I *really* had to like *arduously* calm myself down. And like really set my intention to move ba::ckwards=

Julia: And to almost to like even in fact like try to be a receptive=

Barbara: yeah

Julia: =you know, rather than just being in neutral, [to try and balance myself out.]

Barbara: [yeah, you need to receive] yeah.

Julia: And um, you know, I was able, you know, to varying degrees to sort of coax it out. But I, I felt very self-conscious of that (0.8) that aspect of my personality that I'm learning more and more is this very *physical* reality, and I'm not—

Again, during this segment, the teacher nods and overlaps Julia's speech with approbatory comments, finally choosing to interrupt her student with the following:

Barbara: —Well let me tell you something in your defense, most of us are who drawn to this medicine are drawn because we have a desire to fix things. (3.0) ((nods)) So, you know, the mantra is I'm not a bad person because I can't fix things. ((class laughs)) I'm not a bad person because I can't fix things. I'm not a bad person 'cause I can't fix things. (0.8) You know? That's—we wanna help, we want to make a difference, we want people to feel better. (0.7) Right? So if we can see where the problem is, we're going to be attracted to that(.) But it's not about the problem. It's about the person who has the problem, and in order to do that, you have to receive them, and give validation to their experience. You can't do that if you're overly focused on the problem. (1.5) So good for you for getting it, (.) and good for you for working on it.

With this, the class continues with their sharing.

In these segments, there is a lot going on. To understand what I mean with this, some relatively detailed background is necessary. The following sections thus broadly cover the history of Chinese medicine in China and the West as well as the moral and material landscapes of Chinese medicine in the contemporary United States, emphasizing the unevenness of the terrain, the tensions that permeate the multiple historical and contemporary projects of authenticating Chinese medicine, and the multiple ways in which this unevenness and tension mediates the ways in which the objects of Chinese medicine are understood and utilized.

Chinese Medicine in China: Historical and Institutional Practices

This section describes some of the history of Chinese medicine in China, beginning with an examination of the ways in which the body was traditionally understood and tracking the changes in these understandings in the nineteenth and twentieth centuries. It also very broadly traces the development of multiple forms of diagnosis and treatment in the diverse practices that have emerged as Chinese medicine has become increasingly standardized and institutionalized in the last one hundred years, especially in relation to biomedicine.

Historically, representations of the body in Chinese medicine have never been singular. In other words, there is not now nor has there ever been one Chinese medical body whose characteristics are described, pictured, and explained consistently either within or across texts. Instead, as Farquhar explains, "the Chinese medical body is a multiplicity" (1994: 78). Scheid echoes this by suggesting that "plurality in Chinese medicine commences at the most fundamental level, that of the description and organization of body structure and function" (2002: 27). This multiplicity, or plurality, he suggests, is inherent in the very language that classical Chinese medicine uses to describe the body, as "no single term in classical Chinese corresponds to the English 'body,' with its implicit meaning … of a vat or container and its categorical opposition to 'mind'" (Scheid 2002: 27–28). In a series of rich metaphors, Larré, Schatz, and Rochat de a Vallée (1986) explain the various terms that are used to represent the body in the language of Chinese medical theory, including 形 *xing*, which "presents the body in terms of the 'corporeal form,' the 'appearance' which can be seen and touched," 体 *ti*, which "expresses these organizing principles which structure and unify the body and permit coordination of function and conduct of life," and 身 *shen*, which represents "the entirety of [the] being, which cannot be designated as either material or spiritual … and which causes each person to exist in an individualized way, to unfold his or her life, to take responsibilities, and to act" (Larré, Schatz, and Rochat de a Vallée 1986: 107–108). From this description, plurality is observable as a collection of different perspectives on both the form and meaning of the body in Chinese medicine. As "bodies," then, humans were (and are) approached by physicians of Chinese medicine as composites or "ensemble of the forces, or breaths, that act within the human being and encompass feelings, mores and situations" (Larré,

Schatz, and Rochat de a Vallée 1986: 108). Not just "form," nor simply "function," bodies in Chinese medicine are inherently multiple.

As strange and impractical as this may seem from a biomedical perspective, physicians in China historically developed an intricate system of diagnosis and treatment that depended on an understanding of human bodies as "sites of temporal disjunction, ruptures in cosmic time" (Kuriyama 1994: 31). In contrast to the understanding of the body as a "discrete entity and isolated object" that can be apprehended through dissection and mapping of physical structures and can be diagnosed and treated accordingly (Kuriyama 1999: 262), this meant that diseased bodies in classical Chinese medicine were understood to express a disharmony occurring somewhere between the flow of the seasons, the direction of winds, a person's lifestyle, and the coursing of *qi*, often translated as "energy" or "life force," in the human body (Kuriyama 1994, 1999). The state or condition of a person's *qi* was mapped especially through close observation of pulses and coloring (of the skin, tongue, and eyes). At least after the "medicine of systematic correspondence" came together in the Han dynasty (206 BC–AD 8) findings were interpreted within the frameworks of the five-phase doctrine, which tracks the organic relationships between five interrelated phases of nature, and *yin-yang* theory, which emphasizes the dual opposing and yet complementary forces operating in all phenomena (Unschuld 1985).

It is furthermore important to note here that although *qi*, *yin-yang*, and the five phases existed as relatively unifying theories, individual physicians in China prior to the late nineteenth and early twentieth centuries practiced within their own "lineages," or "currents," as Scheid (2007) calls them. These currents are consistent with each other in that they all draw upon roughly the same set of classical texts and yet differ in the broad-ranging conclusions and forms of practice that emerge from different teachers' interpretations of these texts over time. Unschuld (1985, 2009) thus notes that, although there have been significant and acrimonious debates within the field of medicine in China, seemingly inconsistent theories and practices have existed somewhat harmoniously alongside each other. Andrews describes this diversity in terms of traditional educational models, writing that "for a literate Chinese physician, medical authority rested ultimately on the correct interpretation of the ancient canonical works, as mediated by the teacher" (1996: 178). Pointing to the fact that this mediation occurred through a "vertical transmission from teacher to pupil that was closely modeled on family structures and was often superimposed on them," Andrews further emphasizes that "the considerable variation both within and between these texts allowed for a variety of different approaches to etiology and therapy, and also for significant innovations" (1996: 178). The multiplicity of the body itself was thus mirrored in the diversity of practices characterizing Chinese medicine throughout most of history.

In the late nineteenth and early twentieth centuries in China, multiple social, historical, and cultural circumstances combined to form the need for a more unified system of officially and institutionally recognized "Chinese" medicine. I place "Chinese" in quotes here to emphasize that this system was, in multiple ways, formed in distinct opposition to "Western" medicine, including Western anatomy, Western surgery, and Western forms of diagnosis (Andrews 1996, Karchmer 2004). In this sense, Chinese medicine formulated its identity as a single system (albeit still with multiple, articulating parts) in relation to the medicine of the West. As Western versions of anatomy became more accepted during the late nineteenth and early twentieth centuries, then, physicians of traditional medicine in China realized that "they would have to invent new kinds of truth claims about Chinese medicine" (Karchmer 2004: 75–76). Compromises were made to make the two seem complementary. Overlaps were found and emphasized. Differences were reframed. This was not always an easy process, especially given the diversity in ways of apprehending and treating bodies in historical Chinese medical practices. Thus began efforts to "Orientalize" the body, a process so-named by Karchmer (2004) that included the construction of the Chinese medical body as an entity that was simultaneously distinct from and yet completely compatible with the Western medical body.

Perhaps the most prominent result of this battle was the development and articulation of the "structure-function dichotomy" (Karchmer 2004), where, in opposition to the Western medical body's focus on structure, the Chinese medical body came to represent function:

> The truth of Western medicine was grounded in its detailed knowledge of the anatomical structures of the body, on the primacy of the substrate. The truth of Chinese medicine was based on a different body that emphasized the dynamic and temporal processes of *qi* transformation and the four seasons (Karchmer 2004: 88).

In this vision, the Chinese medical body was conceived as the direct opposite and yet the perfect complement to the Western medical body. Nowhere is this more observable than in the translation of the bodily organs, which prior to the early twentieth century were considered to refer to roughly the same anatomical entities as identified in Western biomedicine (Unschuld 1985; Wiseman 2000c). Within the structure-function dichotomy, however, Western and Chinese body parts are considered to be mostly separate entities. For example, the Western medical heart is considered an organ in the thorax responsible for pumping blood through the organism. The Chinese medical 心 *xin*, or heart, while also responsible for generating the circulation of *xue*, the substance introduced above as "blood" but not blood, is also in charge of "housing" the mind, or *shen*, and "opening" to the tongue in terms of taste and speech, among other things. The implications of this strategic move on the interaction described at the opening of this chapter, when a Western teacher attempts to explain "blood deficiency" vis-à-vis anemia to a Western student, are important to consider and will be examined in detail below. Here, it is important to note very broadly that, within the framework of the structure-function dichotomy, Chinese medical organs, which previously had both functional and structural roles, took on an increasingly functional identity. This move created the space for Chinese medicine to exist side-by-side with biomedicine without threat, as its truth-claims belonged to an entirely different realm.

Here, it is critical to recognize that the unification of Chinese medicine in China was not simply a reactive response to the acceptance of the "superiority" of biomedicine, however. There were also many ways in which the reorganization of Chinese medicine as a coherent system was undertaken as a strategy of resistance, if not to "modernization" per se then to biomedicine and "the West" as a whole (Andrews 1996: 15). Through the appropriation and adoption of (Western) ideas about modernization and progress (see Sinn 2001, Spence 1990), many individuals involved in the creation of Chinese medicine actually worked consciously to implement a modern structure of medicine—a system—that resisted simple "scientization" or "Westernization":

> Chinese physicians mobilized western knowledge as a resource with which to defend themselves and the values they aimed to uphold. In so doing, they appropriated western medical knowledge, so that even though there was much of recognizably western origin in the new Chinese medicine, the Chinese-ness of the end result was never in doubt (Andrews 1996: 2).

Here, Andrews emphasizes the extent to which the distinctive "Chineseness" of Chinese medicine cannot be taken for granted or simplified as a purely politically motivated configuration, a "corrupted" version of traditional forms of medical practice that emerged only as a strategy for coping with the hegemonic forces of biomedicine. Instead, Chinese medicine, in *mobilizing* Western knowledge, created a distinctly Chinese science that capitalized on certain points of overlap with Western medicine without capitulating to the absolute truth-value of this force.

In the 1950s, there was a further push for the delineation of a distinctly "Chinese medical science" that distinguished itself from Western science and yet incorporated the basic principles of scientism in the context of a socialist state (Zhan 2009). At this time, governmental support for Chinese medicine rapidly increased, fueled largely by Mao Zedong's linking of the "treasure-house" of Chinese medical theory to Marxist epistemology (Unschuld 1985: 252). This led to the well-documented invention of "Traditional Chinese Medicine" (TCM). The "immediate goal," writes Zhan, of the state's efforts to support Chinese medicine was to "develop a body of basic theories, which could then be rectified by scientific methods, especially through experiments" (2009: 37).

Thus began serious government-supported efforts to standardize and professionalize Chinese medicine. The resulting paradigm of Traditional Chinese Medicine (TCM), formally taught in newly established institutions of medicine and drawing upon standardized textbooks, was heavily rooted in the structure-function dichotomy, introduced above, where in contrast to biomedical emphasis on structural knowledge and treatment, Chinese medical theory and practice claimed validity in terms of comprehending the functional aspects of the human body. This is the system of official Chinese medicine still in place in contemporary China, where multiple forms of "integrative Chinese and Western medicine" (中西医结合 *zhong xiyi jiehe*) are practiced in hospitals, researched in clinical trials, and discussed in both scholarly and popular formats. Often, the perspectives and practices that emerge from such integrative forms of medicine are quite diverse. So while many lament the loss of traditional knowledge in modernized institutional forms of Chinese medicine, there are also many ways in which the core traditional teachings of Chinese medicine, the many currents of practice that have emerged over centuries among different lines of physicians, still very much exist within the networks of physicians and their students in contemporary China (Scheid 2001, 2007). Many of these individuals practice in hospitals, as well as outside of official institutions.

Chinese Medicine in the United States: Historical and Institutional Practices

Keeping the development of Chinese medicine in China in mind, this section describes the process by which Chinese medicine has grown into an institutionalized, if still peripheral, medical practice in the United States during the twentieth and twenty-first centuries.

Chinese medicine existed in the United States as early as the early nineteenth century, when European experimentations with acupuncture were translated into the medically plural Jacksonian America (Cassedy 1974). As a result of a series of mistranslations in the fifteenth and sixteenth centuries that associated Chinese medical concepts with the outdated Galenic humoral medicine (Barnes 2005a), such "needling practices" were mostly divorced from Chinese philosophical and cultural frameworks. Chinese medicine was also brought to the United States by Chinese immigrants working in the California mining industry in the mid-nineteenth century, when physicians drew upon traditional medical practices to treat everything from mercury poisoning to the common cold (Buell 1998). Other avenues for the transmission of Chinese medicine into the United States include the translation of practices from Japan, Sri Lanka, and Vietnam (Barnes 2013). Likewise, Chinese medicine could be found in some early- to mid-twentieth-century translations from Europe, when individuals such as Soulié de Morant, Paul Nogier, and J. R. Worsley began working to develop more systematic, hybrid theories and applications of acupuncture (Barnes 2013; Eckman 1996; Hsu 1995). Many of these hybrid theories emerged, it is interesting to note, at the same time as thinkers such as Karl Jaspers, Merleau-Ponty, Martin Heidegger, and Carl Jung began turning to Eastern philosophy more seriously to contextualize and complement Western philosophy (Clarke 1997). None of these forms of Chinese medicine really penetrated the mainstream, however, until 1971, when James Reston, the *New York Times* journalist visiting Beijing, wrote an article detailing his experience with acupuncture analgesia during his appendectomy in China.

After Reston's article, a particular set of sociocultural and historical circumstances led to a rapid increase in interest in Chinese medicine. "Instantly, in America," Kao describes, "the word 'acupuncture' was hanging on the lips of many people … there was a great demand for research and information" (1992: 4). Often because of poor study design, most of the funded studies did not produce any significant results. Most physicians were therefore unreceptive to the idea of acupuncture, and the government was reluctant to accept its validity without scientific proof (Kao 1992). Members of the American public, however, were much more curious and open to the idea. "The consumers," writes Kao, "realizing that American medicine with its great advances in recent decades does not harbor all medical knowledge of the world, welcomed the new technology for the treatment of diseases including pain" (1992: 5). The underground practice of acupuncture thus flourished within countercultural circles, as well as by some practicing physicians, many of whom had little more than a weekend of training and tended to rely upon "folk" acupuncturists from Asia for the treatment of patients (Kotarba 1975). While interest in Chinese herbal medicine blossomed later in the development of Chinese medicine in the United States, it is important to note here that the emphasis during this time was on acupuncture only, traditionally considered an adjunct therapy in Chinese medicine (Zhang and Rose 1995).[1]

In the 1970s, the first acupuncture classes, taught mostly by Chinese practitioners, began to spring up in the United States. The texts they used at this time consisted mostly of class notes compiled by students and copied for distribution (Barnes 2003), and most of the students were middle-class Caucasians who saw in acupuncture a "form of protest against biomedicine" (Barnes 2003: 11):

> We were middle class kids, a lot of us. It was illegal as a practice, and we thought we would never make a living at it … It was something of an outlaw role. Having gone through our early adult years as outlaws with a feeling of rejection and of not belonging, we probably outlawed it more than it needed to be. But without outlaws, nothing new comes into the culture (Bob Felt as cited in Barnes 2003: 7–8).

Bob Felt here explains that he and other members of the counterculture who first got involved with acupuncture in the 1970s understood themselves as "outlaws" whose rebellion gave rise to the development of a fresh and new perspective and practice. As Barnes explains, "[T]his process took place in the broader unfolding of what has since come to be called the 'New Age'" (2003: 8), where hippies "sought healthcare that was compatible with its values of egalitarianism, naturalness, mysticism, 'back to the land' philosophy, and vegetarianism" (Baer 2001: 98). Also associated with the New Age "neopagan" or "neoshaman" emphasis on spirituality, many of the 1970s countercultural icons were inspired by images of China as "the China of esoteric wisdom traditions" and "the China of the Maoist revolution" (Barnes 2003: 4), both of which were formed during the years when Westerners had little to no access to China.

Over time, efforts to gain legal status and recognition led to an increased push for the professionalization of acupuncture in the United States:

> As acupuncture gained popular legitimacy, many of the European American practitioners—themselves from middle-class backgrounds—reexamined their cultural role, their identity as practitioners, and their place in the larger cultural field of American medicine. At stake was the question of status and legalization (Barnes 2003: 9).

Because of widespread resistance to the idea of acupuncturists practicing as autonomous physicians in competition with biomedical practitioners, however, most states at first required an MD license to practice acupuncture. Nevada and Oregon were the first states to license acupuncturists in 1973, and in 1978, California was the eighth state to follow suit (acupuncture.ca.gov). By 1979, acupuncturists were recognized as primary health providers in California (Baer et al. 1998). As of 2013, there are forty-four states plus the District of Columbia with acupuncture licensing laws and regulations (nccaom.org/regulatory-affairs/state-licensure-map). No unified national licensure system is in place, however, leaving licensure requirements up to the board of acupuncture or Oriental medicine in each state. Most states at this time require that students pass the national certification exam issued by the National Certification Commission for Acupuncture and Oriental Medicine (NCCAOM), established in 1982. Some states also issue their own state board exam, including California, where students are required to pass the markedly more difficult state exam to practice. As of 2013, the number of acupuncturists in the United States is estimated at about eighteen thousand, with over 50 percent in either California or New York (acufinder.com/Acupuncture+Faqs).

As more states began to recognize and license acupuncturists, the number of acupuncture schools in the United States increased. The 1982 formation of the Accreditation Commission for Acupuncture and Oriental Medicine

(ACAOM) and the Council of Colleges of Acupuncture and Oriental Medicine (CCAOM), officially recognized by the national government in 1990, further fueled this growth. At present, there are more than sixty-five schools of Chinese or "Oriental" medicine in the United States, more than ten of which are in California. Most schools offer a master's degree in Oriental Medicine, which is comprised of about four thousand hours of training. At the present time, most of the acupuncture schools are run as for-profit institutions, but students are generally eligible for Title IV federal financial aid, with an average cost of education running around thirty-thousand dollars for three to four years.

As Barnes explains, "[A] standardized American version of PRC-TCM remains the dominant system of Chinese acupuncture taught in the United States" (2003: 5). Curricula are therefore broken up into about thirty-four hundred hours of Oriental medical study and practice as an intern, and six hundred hours of biomedical study, including chemistry, physics, anatomy, physiology, and pathology. Rarely, some Chinese language is required, usually only a semester. Only a few schools in the United States require Chinese throughout the program.

Although there are increasing numbers of texts available, most schools draw heavily upon three to five required textbooks. One of these, *Chinese Acupuncture and Moxibustion* (Chen 2005), was originally "compiled" under the supervision of the Chinese Ministry of Public Health in 1987 and is loosely based on the required, highly biomedically oriented texts in Chinese programs. Other required texts, for example *Foundations of Chinese Medicine* (Maciocia 2005), *Materia Medica* (Bensky and Gamble 1993; Bensky, Clavey, and Stöger 2004), and *Formulas & Strategies* (Bensky and Barolet 1990; Scheid et al. 2009), are written by Western authors who also use a compilation approach to translation, including some translated material from various Chinese texts, as well as case reports and clinical insights from their own practice. National and state exams are based mostly on these texts (Barnes 2003: 10), and school curricula are tailored to teaching for the tests.

In the contemporary United States, there is also a widespread presence of alternate forms of acupuncture and Chinese medicine, including French energetic lineages, Five-Element Acupuncture, and various forms of "classical" Chinese medicine argued by many to be more authentic than the TCM taught in mainstream schools. The availability of these alternate forms in postgraduate programs, seminars, and multiyear programs ensures that Chinese medical education in the United States is actually quite diverse. Since 2007, the "Doctor of Acupuncture and Oriental Medicine" (DAOM) degree has been approved, and currently five schools in the United States offer two-year doctoral programs for graduates of master's programs. The doctoral programs variably focus on integrative medicine, classical medicine, and specialty practice. Many more schools are currently in the process of applying for DAOM accreditation, and there is also talk in the community about the development of a "first-professional doctorate," which will transform all master's programs into doctoral programs and will add an additional two years of study to the course.

Upon graduation from these institutions, many students seek to establish private practices, with fees ranging from around fifty to one hundred dollars per treatment, plus the cost of herbs. As more conclusive research is published as to the effectiveness of acupuncture and herbal medicine for the treatment of common conditions such as arthritis, headache pain, and back pain, increasing numbers of hospitals and biomedical clinics are incorporating Chinese medicine. Many graduates of Chinese medical schools work in such integrative settings. There is currently a great deal of debate in the acupuncture and Chinese medicine community, however, about what types of sacrifices members need to make to be accepted by the mainstream biomedical health industry. It should also be noted here that an oft-quoted yet not entirely confirmed statistic claims that only about 50 percent of Oriental medicine school graduates are successful in establishing an active practice.

Although institutionalized schooling has indeed become the primary avenue to practice in the contemporary United States, there remain two other significant options. Certain ethnic and community-based practitioners can be "grandfathered in" to the practice of Chinese medicine if they can prove that their educational experience is equivalent to U.S. programs and can pass exams. Likewise, biomedical physicians can participate in a three-hundred-hour certification course to be able to practice acupuncture under the American Board of Medical Acupuncture. Similarly, an increasing number of biomedical schools are offering short courses and internships in acupuncture therapy. Given these different avenues to practice, Marian Katz identifies three main subgroups of practitioners of acupuncture and Chinese medicine in the United States: "ethnic-community-based practitioners," "graduates of American schools of Chinese or Oriental Medicine," and "Medical Acupuncturists." (2011: 35). Unfortunately, there is not a great deal of overlap between these communities in the United States. Like Katz's study, the current study focuses on the subpopulation directly involved with American schools of Chinese or Oriental medicine, including some graduates but also students, teachers, and translators.

Contemporary U.S. Chinese Medicine: Moral Goods

Multiple tensions characterize the identity of the particular subpopulation of persons who are currently involved with or who are products of American schools of Chinese medicine. This section describes several of these tensions in the context of the "goods" informing peoples' interest in and practice of

Chinese medicine. The section thus includes a discussion of the morality of alternative medicine and the moral implications of practicing a medicine understood in contrast to biomedicine in contemporary clinical contexts. Beginning with a general overview of the complementary and alternative medicine (CAM) movement, the section then focuses more specifically on the moral landscape of Chinese medicine in the United States.

As part of the medical counterculture, Chinese medicine in the contemporary United States exists as part of the much broader CAM movement. Even calling this complex trend in medicine a "movement" may be misleading, as there are many modalities encompassed by the label "CAM"—including naturopathy, homeopathy, chiropractic, reiki, and other "energy medicines" (Cassidy 2004)—practiced by individuals who often find fault with being grouped together. Likewise, medical pluralism in the United States is far from a new thing (Baer 1995; Kaptchuk and Eisenberg 2001). Nevertheless, anthropologists, historians, and sociologists, among others, have found it useful, when considering a certain kind of thinking about health, healing, the self, and the body that has emerged over the last fifty years or so in the West, to maintain a wide frame of reference for understanding CAM as a particular movement with a set of core underlying values. As briefly mentioned above in relation to Chinese medicine, the historical roots of CAM more generally lie in the countercultural movements of the 1960s, including the "back to nature" philosophies that contributed to the development of ecological environmentalism and health-food culture (Baer 2004; Barcan 2011). CAM also overlaps with the development of humanistic psychology and the popularity of many self-oriented practices in the West, including psychiatry and psychoanalysis (Baer 2004; Barcan 2011). As mentioned above in the context of the rising popularity of Chinese medicine in the 1970s, CAM generally also has roots in the New Age movement, which emphasizes a self-oriented and perennial spiritual approach to living (Heelas 1996). Feminism, natural birthing, and women's roles in advocating a "gentler and kinder form of healthcare" (Baer 2004: 8) also contributed to the development of CAM. Finally, Barcan also notes the importance of the "health and fitness boom of the 1980s" along with "the continued rise of consumer culture and the globalization of particular healing practices" (2011: 6) as contributing, sometimes more and sometimes less, to the development and rising popularity of CAM. All of these movements, in many ways, have grown out of and have also contributed to a widespread cultural dissatisfaction, especially with biomedicine:

> The increasing popularity of complementary and alternative medicine reflects changing needs and values in modern society in general. This includes a rise in prevalence of chronic disease, an increase in public access to worldwide health in-

> formation, reduced tolerance for paternalism, an increased sense of entitlement to a quality life, declining faith that scientific breakthroughs will have relevance for the personal treatment of disease, and an increased interest in spiritualism. In addition, concern about the adverse effects and escalating costs of conventional healthcare are fueling the search for alternative approaches (Jonas 1998: 1616).

In many ways, then, the CAM movement can be seen as a critique of biomedicine, but also a deep-seated reevaluation of modernity, authority, corporate culture, and science more generally. Even within biomedical circles today, this distinctly moral perspective is gaining a stronger foothold, especially in mainstream medical school programs that are seeking to integrate education in personal awareness and training in various CAM therapies (Charon 2001; Dobie 2007; Elder et al. 2007; Graham-Pole 2001; Greaves 2002; Kligler et al. 2004; Novack et al. 1999).

CAM therapies, generally speaking, are most often understood in terms of a set of distinct qualities. First, most modalities in CAM emphasize a certain form of holism. Holism in CAM is represented in multiple ways, but is often denoted with the recognition of the interconnection between mind, body, and spirit (Goldstein 1999; Ho 2007; McGuire 1988). Spirituality is thus a crucial component of most forms of CAM, especially the notion of a nondenominational "spirit" that "transcends scientific rationalism" (Greaves 2002: 84; see also Brown 1997; Heelas et al. 2005). Within CAM, there is likewise a focus on energy, often described in metaphors of electricity or nature. CAM modalities are thus often conceptualized as working through the "transmission," "balancing," or "releasing" of energy in order to facilitate balance in the body (McGuire 1988: 173–175). Illness, in this formulation, is imagined to be an expression of disharmony. Related to this kind of energetic work, there is also a distinct ambivalence about language in CAM that often generates an overall distrust of "intellectual" engagement with texts and instead supports a reliance upon intuitive practice. This kind of intuitive practice indexes an emerging "ethic of care" in CAM, where there is an emphasis on healing as opposed to curing. In contrast to curing, which "aims at eliminating specific conditions or harm … healing aims to restore wellness or balance to the person as a whole, including the social fabric unraveled by loss, conflict or distress, not just the individual body or part afflicted with misfortune or disease" (Ross 2012: 20). This kind of healing, it is worth noting, is often understood in CAM as a "cooperative process" where "the healer is a partner or a guide, not an omnipotent distant authority figure" (Goldstein 1999: 64), although this process does often involve a sometimes elaborate authoritative performance by the healer (McGuire 1988). It also emphasizes the need for an equal relationship between practitioner and client. Healing emerges from an engaged, resonant relationship with patients that is often considered as a kind of "partnership" (Katz 2011), wherein "a cure always entails commitment on the part of the individual" (Goldstein 1999: 64). CAM therapies further emphasize their use of natural methods that are also described as organic or low-technology, descriptions which are seen to underscore their link to traditional modes of living and healing. Finally, in CAM, it is also important to note, *things* take on an important role, especially in the context of aesthetics. As Barcan 2011 describes it, "Spirituality-in-the-body also chimes with a consumer culture in which inner states are increasingly bound up with commodities ... in particular, they are bound up in the aestheticization of everyday life and the appeal to the senses increasingly offered by the market" (Barcan 2011: 36). Different forms of CAM may emphasize one or more of these qualities over others.

Based on these qualities, CAM is often understood to stand in stark moral opposition to biomedicine. For example, holism is commonly held in contrast to Cartesian dualism and biomedical reductionism (Goldstein 1999). CAM's focus on energy is opposed to biomedicine's emphasis on the physical properties of the body, thereby rejecting "the 'objective' and physically knowable world as the sole locus of the source of the illness" (Goldstein 1999: 14). CAM's naturalness is similarly distinguished from biomedicine's "artificiality," it's "pureness" from biomedicine's "toxicity," its "organic" methods and materials from biomedicine's "synthetic" ones, and its "low-technology" from biomedicine's "high-technology" (Kaptchuk and Eisenberg 1998: 1061–1062). Likewise, tradition in CAM is conceived of in opposition to biomedicine's modernity, and CAM's emphasis on spirituality is held up as an alternative to the science of biomedicine. Personal responsibility and empathic relationships, furthermore, are contrasted with the model of the passive patient and the authoritative doctor in biomedicine, where healthcare has too often come to seem like an economic rather than humanistic interaction (Goldstein 1999: 27). Although many scholars have become resistant to the idea of CAM as alternative or contrary to a reified dominant biomedicine (Wardwell 1994), Katz points out that "removing categorical distinctions between biomedicine and CAM itself obscures the fact that these categories, and the discourses they invoke, have themselves become 'actors' in the construction of medical knowledge and medical practice" (2011: 6). Instead, she notes that "oppositional discourse is found to be part of the warp and weft of the lived understandings and identity constructions of patients and practitioners" (2011: 6). In other words, regardless of the "objective" truth-value of such oppositional claims, the fact that people draw heavily upon them in their understandings of CAM vis-à-vis biomedicine underscores their importance for examining CAM as a frame of thinking about the world of healing.

Clearly, CAM is far from being "just" a medical movement. Several anthropologists and historians have demonstrated that it is also a cultural practice with widespread moral implications. "Alternative therapies are not just purely medical techniques; they are an increasingly popular new form of *cultural practice* bound up in new forms of bodily understanding and perception and new conceptions of selfhood" (Barcan 2011: 2). Many hardcore CAM adherents therefore often identify with one or more counter-cultural movements and/or increasingly mainstream personal ideologies of self-transformation, self-awareness, and self-esteem. Within the moral framework of CAM, one thus finds a search for a more complete or holistic way of understanding the self. Against the backdrop of a biomedical self imagined to be comprised solely of the physical form, this search often focuses intensely on the distinctly Western notion of the self as an interior space of feeling, spiritual experience, and opportunity for reflexive self-transformation (Parish 2008; Taylor 1989). As a reflection of the broader Western "subjective turn" (Heelas et al. 2005), the CAM movement in general further espouses the notions of personal responsibility and self-awareness. In CAM, there is also a special emphasis on the healing of emotional and spiritual imbalances as underlying causes and expressions of physical disorders (Barcan 2011; English-Lueck 1990; Goldstein 1999; Heelas 1996; McGuire 1988; Ross 2012). This is a moral ideal, where healing, notes Heelas, is conceived of as a spiritual practice of shifting away from a "contaminated mode of being—what we are by virtue of socialization—to that realm which constitutes our authentic nature" (1996: 2). Such beliefs are often cultivated prior to the use or study of CAM practices. Indeed, as McGuire notes, healing in CAM "is typically part of a larger system of beliefs and practices that deals with issue such as moral responsibility, social status, and family or community cohesion" (McGuire 1988: 6). CAM practices, furthermore, offer "an *alternative world image*" (McGuire 1988: 244; italics in original) to their adherents, a sense that something else, something better, is possible. This awareness, when it dawns, often generates a personal sense of responsibility or need to change.

Perhaps not surprisingly, this particular moral framework for understanding the self and the role of medicine in society came up frequently in the present study. Many of the students in the school where I carried out my research, for example, come to Chinese medicine motivated by a deeply personal sense of spiritual and moral "awakening" that drives them to seek something different. This seeking is a search for resonance—a search for the invisible, ineffable—that compels several of these individuals who have been involved in prior careers to change their life direction. Treavor, for example, discusses how he quit his job in a competitive corporate culture—a job that he qualified for only after completing an arduous doctoral degree—after hearing Joseph Campbell on television, talking about spirituality and following one's bliss:

> Campbell said ... When you come to a fork in the road, and you need to make a decision between going one way or another, project yourself mentally down those

> two pathways, and your spirit will tell you, 'if I go this way, I'm going to fall off the beam, and if I go that way I'm going to stay on the beam, and the trick,' he said, 'is to stay on the beam.' And the minute I heard him say that I thought I am so not on the beam, it's not even funny, and I went to work the next day and quit. And then I went to sleep for about six weeks, because I was really tired. And then I got up one day, I said, okay, now I need to figure out what I'm gonna do with the rest of my life.

After this turning point, Treavor reflected on what he wanted and decided that he needed to incorporate more spirituality into his life and to be more in touch with himself. "I need to get in my body more. I need to have closer relationships with people, I need to interact more with people … And it was obvious to me that I needed to go in the direction of healthcare." Treavor eventually found his way to Chinese medicine through massage school, inspired by some basic tongue, pulse, and theory books. When he met Julia in a massage course and heard about her plans to start school, he was "triggered" to join her.

From Treavor's comments, the personal drive to change, experienced as an urgent reality, is apparent. Such desires for transformation are not just about the self, however. Several of the students and many of the teachers in the present study further spoke of wanting to "change the world" with Chinese medicine. Julia, for example, said that "a socio-political want to be engaged with healthcare, or with the bettering of society" inspired her to study Chinese medicine. Sarah, a former model, likewise said that "I knew I wanted to do something where I woke up in the morning and felt that I was not doing something that was totally self-indulgent, where I was actually making a difference, or contributing to humanity at some level." In this sense, the students in this study consider themselves active participants in shaping the future of medicine in the United States. As Flesch puts it, "For many students, acupuncture and Oriental medicine presented itself as an epiphany which they described in terms of everything 'clicking' or coming together" (2010: 74). Despite this, many students come to the profession of Chinese medicine with very little idea of the details of the tradition(s). Tina, an early participant in my study who later transferred to an East Coast school, said that when she started, she had no real ideas about what Chinese medicine actually was. She attributes her strong attraction to Chinese medicine to her felt sense that either her ancestors practiced Chinese medicine or that she herself did so in a past life, saying that "I didn't even know what acupuncture was … I hadn't even had a treatment before I started school. Which is the weirdest thing. But I knew like—it just kind of clicked."

To understand what clicks about Chinese medicine, in particular, rather than other forms of CAM, requires a little more in-depth examination. There are many points of overlap. Like CAM, Chinese medicine's holism, represented most often by a focus "on the whole person in his/her social environment"

(Cassidy 1998b: 193), is often contrasted with biomedicine's "reductionism." Many Western sources thus emphasize the wholeness and connectedness of the person in Chinese medicine, explaining that the Cartesian separation between body, mind, and spirit in biomedicine has never existed in Chinese medical thought. Illness, in this formulation, is imagined to be an expression of disharmony, where "discourse about *balance* and *harmony* [work] to construct a TCM version of health that [focuses] on maintaining proper *balance* energetically as well as environmentally" (Ho 2004: 61). In this formulation, the Chinese medical body is often referred to as a "garden" rather than the "machine" of biomedicine (Beinfield and Korngold 1991). Moreover, like other forms of CAM, the "person" in Chinese medicine, in addition to being a garden-body, is understood as having a mind and a spirit, a self that consists not only of the aches and pains, the deregulated hormones or high blood pressure, but also the thoughts, concerns, desires, feelings, and dreams, as well as the sense of connectedness with a larger whole. Chinese medicine as a system that seamlessly relates these aspects of self to each other as well as to the body speaks directly to the Western desire to understand the self in this way. As Barbara, one of the teachers quoted at the outset of this chapter, explains, "I would say that it—for the first time in my life, I got to see the *completeness* of what it meant to be human. That's what Chinese medicine gave to me."

Likewise, as described above, most CAM therapies employ natural, low technology, and/or traditional forms of healing. The use of plants and minerals, in addition to animal parts, as medicinals in Chinese medicine, as well as the reliance upon non-technologically-oriented techniques of acupuncture and moxibustion, is commonly presented as an indication of its naturalness. This connection to nature is further often portrayed within the framework of tradition, linking the practices of Chinese medicine to a more innocent, intuitive time when primitive peoples understood the body via a connection to the natural rhythms of time. Western Chinese medical practitioners thus regularly profess a deep disdain for the excesses of modern technological society and a longing for a more natural relationship to the earth. Students are drawn to this. Tricia, in her first quarter, explains:

> I'm afraid of chemicals, too. So I decided that Chinese medicine—what I like about Chinese medicine is especially that it really has a history behind it. It's not just homeopathic. It is from that thousands of years—you know, it's *cultural*—they have their own science to back it up since it's based on observation, and deduction … over five thousand years … I just thought Chinese medicine seems very complete … I could relate to it, let's just put it that way.

This statement demonstrates the unique sense of trust that the students have in Chinese medicine. They can relate to it as a natural, nonchemical form of medicine, and yet "it's not just homeopathic"—it has a strong basis in empirical knowledge developed over time. Even better, it is *cultural,* that is to say that it is strongly grounded in a particular culture that is not only ancient, but entirely foreign.

Similarly, like in CAM, which emphasizes healing at the level of "energy," Chinese medicine is centered on the notion of *qi,* understood as the vital energetic source uniting both structural and functional realities of body, mind, and spirit. Translations for *qi,* explored in more depth in chapter 4, include "energy," "life force," and even "prana" (from Ayurveda). Although in Chinese medicine there is much literature emphasizing that *qi* is not just energy, that it constitutes "matter" as well, there is a tendency especially in the West as well as in much of TCM to understand *qi* more in terms of the nonmaterial, functional aspects of the body. For example, the flow of *qi* in the body not only regulates the emotions, but also the mind and the digestive process. "Stagnation" of *qi* causes pain, both physical and emotional. To treat any disorder, moreover, *qi* must be accessed through touch, through needling, or through prescriptions that affect the body. To access or feel *qi,* some argue, one must let go of the scientific preoccupation with visual or linguistic proof (Ho 2004). In a statement that will come up repeatedly over the course of this book, and which we will see echoed in many other student comments, Julia discusses the extent to which she views the nature of *qi* as being beyond language, located more in the felt experience of the body than a word:

> I don't see any reason to try and *force* that into a word that we already have in English. Doesn't seem necessary. It is *qi.* Learn it. It's the *new medicine,* you know, here it is … [Clients] will ask what's *qi*? And I'll be like, aw, *qi*'s kind of like you're universal life force energy—it's all in the *world,* it's coming in you, it's going out of you, it's like, you know, it's makin' things happen, it *is* those things that are happening, like, and it is that *heat* that you are feeling in you ankle right now.

It is here that the notion of *qi* overlaps with the emphasis on intuition and embodied spiritual connection prevalent more generally in CAM. Intuitive practice is, indeed, heavily favored in U.S. Chinese medicine. A fourth-year student intern explains the way he understands the difference between "book learning" and intuitive practice: "Book learning is intellectual," he says, "and intuition is instinctual. And the book learning, I think, is very important—I don't want to discount it. But it's what they can teach you. Intuition is what they can't teach you." Students in U.S. Chinese medicine, as in CAM more generally, are attracted especially to learning that which cannot be taught. This includes an emphasis on the importance of psychological as well as physical well-being, an aspect that requires the practitioner "to work from a kind of embodied experience and embodied knowledge" (Ho 2004: 64). Because of this, students and practitioners of Chinese medicine often emphasize that the practice requires an intuitive approach based on "actual lived experience" (Ho 2004: 64).

To learn that which cannot be taught in Chinese medicine further requires a turn toward the self, and the cultivation of spiritually informed, intuitive skills. In this sense, Chinese medicine in the contemporary United States mirrors the broader subjective turn, and the turn toward a nondenominational spirit referenced above as influential in the wider CAM movement. Julia, in her second quarter, professes a distinct moral commitment to self-reflection and the development of self-understanding as part of her study, saying "everybody has to commit to really look at themselves." She uses the Chinese term 神 *shen,* often translated as "spirit" or "mind," to suggest that it is reflective of a kind of mental or spiritual disturbance to set about practicing Chinese medicine without "some sort of meditative understanding of yourself":

> I mean, what I said before about, you know, that you could have all this information? But if you don't understand it, it's useless. I mean … I think it's almost worse than useless. Like if you tried to apply this information without having like a real physical-energetic understanding of what it means, like it's *dangerous.* It's like—it's wrong. It reflects a serious *shen* disturbance on your own part, if you're even trying to do that. So yeah, I mean, you have to cultivate some sort of meditative understanding of yourself.

Julia's statement here indexes the way in which she views the practice of Chinese medicine as a deeply spiritual endeavor. Sarah agrees with her, saying in her third quarter, "[Y]ou have to understand the spirituality of the medicine." The spirituality that Julia and Sarah refer to here consists in one sense of Daoist as well as some Buddhist spiritual ideas informing the theories and practice of Chinese medicine. Contemporary U.S. students, along with many Westerners in general, are often very inspired by such spiritual foundations, especially their attendant practices of self-cultivation and inner alchemy, meditation and contemplation, and understandings of the flow of time in nature (see Clarke 2000; Coleman 2001).

The spiritual self-cultivation of Chinese medicine resonates with students beyond simply as a prerequisite for understanding the spiritual foundations of the medicine, however. As Julia's statement above demonstrates, it is also understood as a personal, embodied form of spirituality that allows them to show up fully for patients. One teacher explains the mechanics of this, saying that "if you can calm your inner world, you can better dance with somebody's chaotic world over there … you're modeling energy for the patient." Embodied self-spirituality thus also exists as a learned form of embodied morality related to the ethic of care emphasizing partnership and healing, as opposed to curing, also prominent in CAM more generally. Barbara, the teacher quoted in the second vignette presented above, thus explains her perspective on her role as a healer as being facilitative rather than causative: "I mean, in the bigger picture of things, I know I make a difference? But each success, I know, is the patient's success; all I did was make space for it." In her third quarter, Sarah echoes this ethos, saying that "it *is* an *art* as well where you really have to connect with the patient, and draw on as much knowledge as you can to be able to heal that person, or help heal that person—to facilitate healing." In correcting her own statements—moving from an understanding of herself as "healing" to "helping heal" to "facilitating healing," Sarah here provides an insight into the moral shift in thinking about care that happens over the course of studying Chinese medicine in this program. Healing here is seen as emerging out of an engaged, resonant relationship with patients, where patients' own participation is seen as equally important as the providers' efforts. Treavor, in his fourth quarter, explains how he really learns this ethic in his own experience of getting treatments from one of his teachers:

> I think my experience with acupuncture on this issue has been me going into the clinic and saying I'm in this room, I want to be in that room. There is a door. I just need somebody to unlock it. So I can open the door and walk through and go into the next room … Like I'm the one who's in the room, and I'm the one who's gonna walk through that door, and I'm the one who's going to occupy the next space, but getting a little help, you know, open—overcoming the barrier between one space and the next is something that I think acupuncture is brilliant at.

For Treavor, as for Julia and Sarah, experiences in his own body inform the way he understands acupuncture and Chinese medicine more generally. The ethic of participation and mutuality in care in Chinese medicine thus develops as an embodied, often spiritually referenced process of self-discovery.

The moral landscape of Chinese medicine in the United States is thus heavily saturated with the morals and ideals of CAM. The "goods" of holism, self-spirituality, energy, balance, intuition, healing, naturalness, and tradition pervade the process of learning at every juncture. These are deeply felt goods rather than abstract ideals. As I have shown, like in CAM generally, they are experienced as ruptures with the ideals of biomedicine. This oppositional discourse often creates nothing short of a moral battlefield. Here, we witness the moral landscape of Chinese medicine becoming more uneven and more fraught with tension. The "battlefield" thus consists of several shifting moral positions. For example, the wholesale linking of Chinese medicine with the CAM movement has sparked several critiques from medical historians and anthropologists. The linking of Chinese medicine to a natural, holistic, spiritual tradition is, Scheid claims, part of the Western association of Chinese medicine "with romanticist critiques of modernity" (2002: 43). As such, it has often been noted that Chinese medicine offers a whole worldview or ideological perspective, rather than simply a medical practice or technique (Hare 1993; Ho 2004; Unschuld 2003; Wiseman n.d.). This ideology, some claim, can be blinding. For example, because of the tendency for students to seek Chinese medical training in response to a critique of biomedicine, some scholars argue that Westerners' understanding of and appreciation of Chinese medicine is clouded by their understanding of Chinese medicine in terms of what biomedicine *is not* rather than what Chinese medicine *is*, independent of biomedicine (Unschuld 2003; Wiseman 2002b, n.d.). "There is a tendency," Wiseman writes, "to assume that any desirable qualities that Western medicine lacks must be present in Chinese medicine, and to project those qualities into Chinese medicine. In the process of projecting ideas onto Chinese medicine, other features have been obscured" (Wiseman n.d.: 28). Wiseman thus asserts that the Western tendency to interpret Chinese medicine as inherently less reductionistic, more holistic, more natural, more intuitive, more patient-centered, and gentler than biomedicine distorts the truth that Chinese medicine "did not develop to suit the taste of people dissatisfied with Western medicine in the twentieth and twenty-first centuries" (Wiseman n.d.: 4). Although Wiseman admits that Chinese medicine is in some ways "more natural, more holistic, and less alienating if not more caring that modern Western medicine," he emphasizes that the vast repertoire of Chinese medicine also includes many instances of symptom-based, reductionistic, and mechanistic approaches to treatment (Wiseman n.d.: 13). He therefore cautions that "there is sufficient evidence to warn against generalizations when describing either Chinese medicine or modern Western medicine" (Wiseman n.d.:13). The wholesale acceptance of Chinese medicine on these generalized terms, he argues, constructs that are too seldom questioned by those who employ them, propels the Western tendency to disregard the original Chinese medical sources and results in a hampering of proper understanding.

Second, the moral battlefield consists of students' own struggles to make sense of their place in the scheme of contemporary healthcare systems. So while students may be motivated by the self-oriented, embodied, holistic, and spiritual goods of Chinese medicine, once they begin their studies, a major tension often emerges as students are faced with the struggle of legitimating their practice of Chinese medicine in a healthcare environment dominated by biomedicine. Flesch (2010) examines the impact of this struggle on the experience of Chinese medical students in one American program, writing that:

> It struck me during my first quarter in the Clinic that students and supervisors of AOM [Acupuncture and Oriental Medicine] were working under the watchful eye of an Absent Physician, whose presence was keenly felt and whose treatments, diagnoses, and prescriptions must be navigated by students and practitioners of AOM (Flesch 2010: 63).

Flesch further details the many ways in which students feel that they have to learn how to "translate" Chinese medicine into biomedical or scientific terms to succeed in the competitive U.S. healthcare market. Katz (2011) confirms that "as a practical matter, all acupuncturists in the United States are faced with the question of how they are going to orient to biomedicine, including how they are going to manage the biomedical information and perspectives brought in by their patients" (224). Some individuals do engage in what Katz calls a "pragmatist" stance toward biomedicine, encouraging their patients to utilize whatever healing practices work for them and actively making efforts to explain Chinese medicine in scientific terms (Katz 2011: 37–38; see also Flesch 2010). In fact, for many individuals (and for all individuals at certain times), such a stance is not necessarily just strategic, but commonsensical. Here, the seemingly totalizing moral framework of spiritualized Chinese medicine gives way in moments where a clear approach toward relating biomedicine to Chinese medicine seems to burst through the tension that derives from the desire of many students and practitioners to challenge biomedicine. This is often a surprise for the students, especially those who expect complete divergence. For example, Julia, in her first quarter, talks about her excitement and shock when she realizes that a part of the brain, the medulla oblongata, lies underneath a major acupuncture point:

> I think it's like *AMAZING* [laughs] I thought it was *AMAZING*, I mean I told my waiter, I was sitting at like lunch at this café when I, you know, and when I—and I discovered all this, I was like *LOOK AT THIS BOOK and LOOK AT THIS BOOK* and it's *AMAZING* and I don't even—you know? … I mean in *some* ways it's like kinda—like it makes sense, like of *course*. But like what does it like even *MEAN*, you know, and what does that then start to convey about like what we're talking about with these like *energy* levels with the different *depths* and the whole *thing*.

Julia's excitement here is palpable, sparked by the curiosity and exhilaration of the underlying questions about the relationships between the biomedical body and the Chinese medical body and the implication that they are not entirely different. Questions like this come up constantly throughout the four-year program, as students struggle with the various moral ideals of opposition and integration. The opening vignette of this chapter, in fact, included just this type of question in regards to the relationship between anemia and blood deficiency.

That said, there is a very real moral tension as students and practitioners struggle to maintain a separate clinical identity in the face of biomedical hegemony. "Students questioned the 'fairness' of having to change, translate, or prove their medicine in order to accommodate Western practitioners," writes Flesch, "as well as the implications of such translations for the authenticity and identity of TCM" (2010: 187). As Barnes explains, in the early to mid-1990s, the number of required biomedical hours was a subject of intense debate among different contingencies of acupuncturists in the United States where "one contingent asserted that acupuncturists should learn to speak 'biomedicine' well enough to be able to order biomedical tests and read the results" (2003: 15) and the other identified more strongly with the countercultural rejection of anything biomedical. This forced members of the burgeoning acupuncture community to reconsider how they wanted to construct their public image:

> The wars over science course requirements ... pushed practitioners of all schools to look hard at how they wanted to define themselves and at how they wished to be perceived by others. Did they want to be classified as primary care givers defined by intensive training in biomedical science? The subtext, for a significant number of them, was the question of what this classification had to do with their own reasons for going into acupuncture in the first place as well as with their own understanding of, and commitment to, Chinese medicine as a system in its own right (Barnes 2003: 15).

In emphasizing the underlying issues for the school curriculum debate participants, Barnes here demonstrates how tensions in the school index the broader debate surrounding the increased push for professionalization, standardization, and institutionalization of acupuncture in the United States. A relatively large contingent of practitioners thus argues that enhanced biomedical knowledge and heightened professional standards would increase acupuncturists' prestige, encouraging more interest from potentially curious yet conservative patients and promoting more support from insurance companies. An equally large contingent of practitioners and students, however, resist the idea of such conformity, arguing that acupuncturists must not give in or "sell out" to such societal pressures. Katz dubs such resistors as "purists":

> Purists argue that their "purer," and thus more "authentic," approach to Chinese medicine offers the best clinical results for patients. Often highly critical of biomedicine, they look to the past, to a time prior to biomedicine, for information and inspiration (Katz 2011: 37).

In most Chinese medical schools in the United States, then, there is an active and ongoing dialogue about biomedicine: how to contrast it with Chinese medicine, how to provide care that addresses the areas that biomedicine is seen to be lacking in, and how to frame one's practice in a way that will be contrary yet still acceptable. This dialogue indexes the moral tensions that often appear within individuals rather than just between idealized notions of "purists" and "pragmatists." Within the daily process of learning Chinese medicine in the contemporary United States, individuals frequently shift back and forth and often end up somewhere in between. In the present study, students expressed a growing ambivalence toward their increasingly demanding class load in biomedicine, complaining that it took their focus away from the Chinese medical content they wanted to focus on, but agreeing that a certain amount was indeed necessary. In her third quarter, for example, Sarah says, "You know, we have these particular pathologies that have been labeled in a Western culture, and I think we have to be able to integrate that into our practice … even though it's not the pure medicine."

Discussions of "pure" versus pragmatic or integrative forms of Chinese medicine points us toward another aspect of the moral landscape worth examining here. This is a tension unique to Chinese medicine, a tension that links back to Chinese history, the formation of the systematized form of Traditional Chinese Medicine (TCM), and the popularity of Chinese medicine in the United States as an alternative moral practice. Although school curricula and exams are based upon TCM, there is widespread recognition that TCM was compiled as a Communist solution to particular political and social ills. Students interpret this medicine as a corruption of the true traditional, spiritually informed classical Chinese medicine. "The narrative of TCM's inauthenticity," writes Van Hoy "is a powerful magnetizing influence in the community of Chinese medicine in the United States" (2010: 77). In her third quarter, Sarah explains what this narrative means to her:

> I think a lot of the texts that are being translated now are TCM, which is you know, just the *communist* kind of *idea* where they have stripped down a lot of the art, and they have stripped down a lot of the old concepts from the medicine to make it more Westernized, and more appealing to Western thought … Because, you know, for *fear* that we won't understand it, and [fear that we will] therefore write Chinese medicine off as something that is not … scientifically based … whereas, you know, you look at classical Chinese medicine, that actually does go further back to study more of the culture, um (pause)—you know, I think that a lot of those texts still aren't being translated, so to be able to have access to that, and access to the older part of this medicine, and the origins of it, and understand more where it came from—why, *why* it has evolved the way it has over several thousands of years—not just what it's been stripped down to in the last fifty years.

As it is this spirituality and depth that the students claim to want most, seeking out the so-called real Chinese medicine has become a deeply personal project for many current U.S. students and practitioners. For some of these folks, it has become a project of searching for what Jay, Mei Zhan's American informant, described as "the little old lady in some rural village deep in China who does *real* Chinese medicine" (Zhan 2002: 186). As Zhan points out, this search directly indexes "an essentialist desire for the truly primordial and authentic—a desire with distinctive old-school Orientalist overtones" (Zhan 2002: 186; see also Said 1979 for a discussion of "Orientalism"). For others, the perceived inauthenticity of TCM as an "invented tradition" (Hobsbawn and Ranger 1983) or a McDonaldization of Chinese medicine encourages them to examine alternative forms, such as J. R. Worsley's Five-Element system or the energetic acupuncture of Mark Seem. In recent years, practitioners translating "classical" Chinese medicine, including Jeffrey Yuen and Heiner Fruehauf, among others, have also become increasingly popular. Although many of these teachers have created a distinctly Westernized version of classical Chinese medicine, several work hard to maintain a connection with alternative currents in China (Scheid 2007).

The search, even for "purists," is thus not just a search for historically or linguistically authentic forms. As Van Hoy points out, it is also a search for a language and form of Chinese medicine that resonates with particular notions and experiences of personhood:

> The discovery of a real Chinese medicine is often tethered to the ability of the medicine to access the rich, inner life of the individual. TCM is not seen to access or address this inner reality. With a handful of terms like stagnation, heat, dryness, deficiency, and phlegm, TCM is not able to articulate the nuances of interpersonal and affective experiences (Van Hoy 2010: 91).

In this view, TCM is almost as bad as biomedicine in terms of being linguistically and culturally void of the types of knowledge-forms that are needed to address the kinds of imbalances that arise in the deep self as experienced by Western individuals. These imbalances include feelings of loss of self-purpose, apathy, and isolation, among others. While not all teachers and authors working on the translation of Chinese medicine into English capitulate to these desires (one Chinese teacher in the school where I conducted research, for example, complained about the tendency for his students to view Chinese medicine as a religion), classical forms of Chinese medicine, as interpreted by contemporary "Masters" such as Jeffrey Yuen and Lonny Jarrett, appeal much more broadly in this sense. Yuen, for example, who does not publish texts but only offers in-person seminars, speaks often of the esoteric implications of points and medicinals. His lectures are full of ideas of how Chinese medical alchemy can be used to treat personality disorders, blocked creativity, low self-esteem, "inability to evolve," and so forth. Jarrett, who I examine in more depth in chapter 3, also speaks of using classical wisdom to access one's own and one's patient's authentic Self.

There are several other examples of teachings that formulate links between contemporary issues of the deep self and classical Chinese medicine, including the writings of Ted Kaptchuk, Mark Seem, Harriet Beinfield and Efram Korngold, Lorie Dechar, and others. A key feature of most of these interpretations, however, is the layering of "language deriving from psychotherapy" (Barnes 1998: 416), as well as contemporary spirituality into the translations. As such,

Chinese medicine is drawn upon in the "aesthetic project" of "therapeutic self-fashioning" (Van Hoy 2010: 129), and it quickly becomes a moral project of trying to find an authentic Chinese medical practice that accesses the "depths" of authentic self (see also Pritzker 2012c). Van Hoy, based on her own experience as a practitioner, contrasts the kind of authenticity that is to be found in these "psychologized" (Barnes 1998) or Westernized forms, to that of a more historical nature:

> I have encountered and studied many of these systems in the course of my training as an acupuncturist. Many of them do seem to provide access to an inner meaning and nuance that TCM fails to be able to articulate. Clearly, such access to a zone of depth and meaning does not automatically make a style of practice more authentic in historical terms. However, such access does have the effect—it does the work—of authenticating practice. Practitioners organize clinical knowledge differently based on this learning. They make diagnoses, choose acupuncture points, and design herbal formulas in ways that reflect personal commitments to authenticity and depth (Van Hoy 2010: 93).

Here, Van Hoy highlights the cultural validity of hybrid forms of Chinese medicine. As she does, she emphasizes the moral force of such practices in the "culture of authenticity" (Lindholm 2008; Taylor 1989, 1991) that places a great deal of importance upon authentic selves:

> This is the powerful moral ideal that has come down to us. It accords crucial moral importance to a kind of contact with myself, with my own inner nature, which it sees as in danger of being lost, partly through the pressures towards outward conformity, but also because in taking an instrumental stance to myself, I may have lost the capacity to listen to this inner voice. And then it greatly increases the importance of this self-contact by introducing the principle of originality: each of our voices has something of its own to say … Being true to myself means being true to my own originality, and that is something only I can articulate and discover. This is the background that gives moral force to the culture of authenticity (Taylor 1991: 29).

Such concerns cut to the very core of what it means to be a person in the world and create tensions within students and practitioners of Chinese medicine who seek something beyond what they find in either TCM or biomedicine. Indeed, as described above, it is often a turning toward the self that ultimately informs the practices that emerge out of this kind of tension. Again, however, this self-oriented strategy for engaging with Chinese medicine meets resistance from scholars who question the ways in which "the medicine" is drawn upon as a moral framework for answering the types of questions one traditionally finds answered in religion (Unschuld 2009: 202–203). The multiplicity of perspectives on this issue, as well as the issue of how Chinese medicine ultimately relates to biomedicine and other forms of CAM, demonstrates the diversity and complexity of the moral landscape surrounding Chinese medicine in the contemporary United States, a landscape that serves as major mediating force in any translation. This section has, very broadly, provided the major contours of this landscape.

Contemporary U.S. Chinese Medicine: Material Goods

Before I return to a discussion of the ethnographic vignettes that opened this chapter, this short section ventures into the complex terrain of materiality, looking at the objects that are made and remade in the translation, teaching, and practice of Chinese medicine in the contemporary United States. Books have already come up several times in this chapter—required textbooks as well as alternative, spiritually oriented texts. As objects, it is perhaps easy to see the ways in which books constitute an enactment of translation in Chinese medicine and the way they might constantly mediate this enactment through both their production and consumption. Further chapters enter into a deeper analysis of this. Here, I want to shift the focus, if briefly, to the other kinds of objects in Chinese medicine. These objects, I suggest, play an important role in the mediation of translation, especially in the context of aesthetics and morality. In particular, I want to look at acupuncture needles. There are many other objects in Chinese medicine. There are white coats that students must put on to legitimate their practice in the school clinic. There are the herbs and other medicinal substances that students learn, imbibe, and prescribe. There are also the crystals and essential oils that interns bring to augment their patients' experience. By looking at acupuncture needles here, I do not intend to discount these other objects. As an example of the ways in which objects mediate the enactment of translation of morality into practice, through the very real interface between practitioners and bodies, acupuncture needles serve here merely as a window in the role that objects can play in the mediation of translation.

"Today's acupuncture needles, tailored to Western sensibilities, are coated with silicone," writes Unschuld (2009: 213). In the context of his 2009 book, I would say that here he is metaphorically highlighting the ways in which Western appropriations of Chinese medicine create a top-coat or protective layer—of morals, desires, demands—around Chinese medicine, one that often has nothing to do with Chinese medicine in China, or at least very little. I discussed this above. Here, I want to look at the nonmetaphorical nature of Unschuld's statement. It points to the ways in which the "sensibilities" of Western participants are mapped onto the physical forms of Chinese medicine here, as silicone coating on disposable acupuncture needles. Historically, of course, acupuncture needles were not made with silicone, nor were they disposable. The point is not about acupuncture needles per se, however, but about the ways in which needles—or any of the material objects in Chinese medicine—participate in the enactment of it, how they make Chinese medicine what it is.

This came up frequently in my study. The students are not unaware of the extent to which their "stuff" will be a participant in the shaping of their new identity as a practitioner of Chinese medicine. Sarah sums it up perfectly when, on the first day of her needling class, she talks about her excitement about going out "on a shopping spree" with Julia to buy the things she needs for her needling kit—needles, cotton balls, hand sanitizer, alcohol swabs, and a sharps container for needle disposal. "I'm more excited than I am about going shopping for shoes or handbags!" she says. The things included in the needling kit can be understood as indices of the kinds of relationships Sarah will form with her future clients. In the West, we recall, this relationship is about connection, continuity, reciprocity, and depth. It is a partnership that distinguishes itself from the relationship between a biomedical practitioner and her patient. The role that needles specifically play in this relationship is demonstrated by Anderson (2010) when he describes an interaction between an acupuncturist and her patient:

> Heidi proceeds to insert several needles while asking Anna if she can feel them, to which Anna acknowledges with both verbal and non-verbal (e.g., nodding) affirmations. After she has inserted one into Anna's upper chest, Heidi asks if she can feel it. Anna's response is slow, but affirmative. Heidi then says, "Now we're waiting for the *qi* to arise, so you end up feeling a sort of electricity going through you." With each insertion Heidi again asks if Anna can feel it. Anna continues with her nonverbal, affirmative responses (Anderson 2010: 262).

In this excerpt, Heidi, the acupuncturist, constantly communicates with Anna, her patient. The rapport between them is not something that is established in the beginning of the session, only to be abandoned when the patient lies passively on the table. It continues in the insertion of each needle. It is nonverbal, affective, and sustained. It is a particular form of interaction that indexes the moral frameworks in which Heidi and Anna find themselves together as practitioner and patient. In the last section, I discussed the ways in which these moral frameworks shape the desire of Western students to become practitioners of Chinese medicine, as well as the way they interpret the material.

Engagement with objects like needles is not something that comes naturally for the students, however. They have never worked with such things before and often are quite fearful of using them to penetrate the bodies of their future patients. As they talk to their teacher as well as to each other (and sometimes to me) over the course of their one-quarter Needling I course, the students reveal some of these fears. While she is needling Sarah for the first time, Julia talks about her fears to her teacher: "For me, there's a big fear that I'm gonna hit something when I thrust." Her teacher responds by saying that this is a healthy fear, a fear that can be managed with a firm understanding of the physiology, particularly the vasculature, arteries, and nerves at the points. On a more "energetic" level, it also needs to be managed through a firm commitment to feeling where the *qi* is before needling, as well as a constant interaction and monitoring of the patient's body. "Because a lot of patients won't be expressive, you have to pay attention ... it's like driving and looking in the rearview mirror at the same time." The moral demands of connection, partnership, and spiritual commitment are embodied in such direction. To accomplish this, the teacher reminds the students, they must be able to "ground" or center themselves in their own bodies, their own self-spirituality, first. Julia thus also talks about her "conversation" with Sarah's body, as felt through the needles as well as in her pulse, which Julia repeatedly checks over the course of the treatment. After the first needle is inserted, for example, Julia says, "I felt the *qi*—it grabbed [the needle]." She then feels Sarah's pulse again, saying, "It's funny, I hear her pulse saying ok, ok ... I feel the impact ... heck, I feel the conversation. There's so much here with the teaching, that she knows it's my first time."

When acupuncture needles—or any other objects—are enacted in the context of such learning, they become more than just objects. They are the vehicles for moral frameworks to find expression in and through action. They are also mediators, I argue, of the ways in which language—words like *qi*, *yin*, or *yang*, pulse terms like "slippery" or "wiry," or even the names of herbs and other substances—gets translated into English. Later chapters demonstrate this process in some detail.

Discussion: Back to Blood and Self-Discovery

From this lengthy digression into history, institutional contexts, moral landscapes, and material goods, we begin to get a sense of some of the complex historical, political, social, and personal processes underlying the interactions described at the outset of this chapter. In the first excerpt, we recall, a student asks her teacher, Carter, about blood deficiency and how it relates to blood volume, or anemia, as understood in biomedicine. This simple question not only indexes but also calls forth decades of searching, in both China and the United States, for parallels between biomedicine and Chinese medicine. As I described in detail above, there are numerous historical, moral, and institutional dimensions to this search and the way it has been resolved in different iterations at different times and in various places. With this one question, then, echoes of the anatomy crisis in early-twentieth-century China can be heard. So, too, echoes of the ongoing morally grounded struggles that students face in the contemporary United States as they strive to reconcile biomedicine and Chinese medicine or other forms of CAM in their own understanding and own practice. The way it is resolved in this particular instance further echoes these struggles and the solutions they have generated in the past.

Carter's response reframes the question in terms of a hypothetical patient interaction, where a patient asks the question about whether they will be automatically diagnosed with blood deficiency if they are anemic, and vice versa. Carter answers his own question (the patient's question) with a firm no and then explains, in both gesture (he interlinks his fingers on both hands) and language, that despite the lack of exact correlation, "there is some crossover ... but there's not a definitive connection." This leads him into a conversation about what "we" mean when we say blood, asking, "Does it include what they're talking about? Is it also something else?" He answers his own question again, with an affirmative, and then goes on to explain the difference:

> What do we mean when we say blood? Does it include what they're talking about? Is it also something else? And the answer is yes (.) um, we are talking about the Western version of blood, but it's also all these additional, you know, concepts associated with the blood in Chinese medicine, so (.) um, the perspective is that we can detect, ah, blood deficiency=what you'd say in Western medicine is subclinical, alright=it's not going to appear on the laboratory test. But our assumption is that left untreated, it ultimately *would,* right? We're just detecting it, um (.) before the test does.

With this response, Carter is enacting the translation of "blood" in Chinese medicine. His words also echo history, especially calling forth early-twentieth-century efforts to redefine Chinese medicine in terms of function, as opposed to biomedical structure. He is enacting, in other words, the structure-function dichotomy, discussed above, and is participating in the collaborative imaginary of Chinese medicine as an insubstantial precursor, the functional that happens before the structural. In history, this framework served a purpose in that it at least superficially resolved, along acceptable lines, the fundamental tension underlying the differences between biomedical and Chinese medical approaches to the human body. Here, the real Chinese medicine was (re)made (and is continually remade in statements like Carter's) as a perfect complement to biomedicine, a precursor to biomedical ways of knowing. Strategic moves made in the early twentieth century in China live on in the distinction that a twenty-first-century American teacher makes for a student who is confused about the difference between the biomedical category of "anemia" and the Chinese medical category "blood deficiency."

In Carter's response there are also echoes of concerns that are unique to the U.S. context of the question. Carter thus invokes the framework of the practitioner-patient dyad that the student will be practicing within. In phrasing his response as a dialogue between these two players, he is teaching students how to talk to patients who are accustomed to the perspectives and vocabulary of biomedicine, drawing upon the use of deictics "we" and "they" to initiate students into a professional role that distinguishes them from patients as well as from biomedical practitioners. In other words, his response both indexes and engenders a certain kind of practice of Chinese medicine—an institutionally accepted form of partnership between practitioner and patient that emerges through detailed explanation, as well as a form of practice that is distinct from biomedicine. As I noted at the outset of this chapter, interactions like this one are quite commonplace in U.S. contexts of learning Chinese medicine.

In the second segment, Julia shares her experience with feeling pulses for the first time. In her share, we learn detailed information about her previous experience with touching patients in her massage practice. We learn, for example, that she tends to go in "too deep too fast," even when clients request her to be softer. We learn that this is a struggle for her, a challenge that she felt in her first attempts at feeling the pulse in class. She talks about a metaphorical "hole" in her partner's pulse. She almost gets sucked into this open space, and has to back herself up in order to "receive" the pulse instead of pushing her own "energy" in. She learns from this that this is a physical reality of her personality. Her teacher, Barbara, encourages her for "working on it," for seeing this about herself. She further relates Julia's tendency to go in too deep and too fast as an expression of the Western student's desire to "want to fix things," to want to find the problem and make a difference. "But it's not about the problem," she says, "it's about the person who has the problem … you have to receive them, to give validation to their experience." She repeats the mantra "I'm not a bad person because I can't fix things" multiple times. The class participates. They laugh.

This exchange, like the first, contains echoes of multiple historical, institutional, and moral realities. The deeply felt desire for embodied knowledge that Julia is seeking, and that she seemingly attains in her discovering of the physical aspects of her personality, resounds with the self-referenced spirituality that many CAM adherents, including many students of Chinese medicine, aspire to. The CAM-wide desire to engage with human bodies in a certain way is also apparent in Julia's efforts to retrain herself to engage with her partner/patient more along the lines of the kind of receptive practitioner that she is seeking to become. Barbara, her teacher, rewards her attempts. In Barbara's response, there is also an implicit comparison of Chinese medicine and biomedicine. Biomedicine is born of a mindset of wanting to fix things, while Chinese medicine is about something different—the functional, yes, but also what comes *with* the functional—the whole person, body-mind-spirit, that which Chinese medicine seeks to receive, and to affect rather than fix.

Conclusion

I have covered a lot in this chapter. History. Institutions. Morality. Objects. Each of these is immensely complex. I do not pretend to have comprehensively examined all of them. If anything, I only touched upon the surface of them in the spirit of offering some background into the very real, deeply felt, embodied, political, and social landscapes that are textured by multiple ways of viewing and experiencing Chinese medicine, language, bodies, or acupuncture needles. These landscapes, I suggest, and the ways in which people engage with them, participate in mediating the enactment of translation in Chinese medicine. The diverse texture of such landscapes, and the ways in which participants shift between them—experiencing themselves and others, bodies and acupuncture needles, books and histories—comprise a large portion of the overlapping grounds upon which living translation unfolds.

Notes

1. Interestingly, the rise in popularity of acupuncture in the United States prompted a similar reaction in China, where acupuncture started to gain more recognition and increasingly became a primary Chinese medical therapy.

CHAPTER

2

Ideas about Words, and Words about Ideas

道可道非常道　*The way that can be spoken is not the constant way*
名可名非常名　*The name that can be named is not the constant name*
无名天地之始　*The nameless was the beginning of heaven and earth*
有名万物之母　*The named was the mother of myriad creatures.*
—Lao Tzu, *Tao Te Ching,* lines 1–4, translation by DC Lau

With the understanding of historical, institutional, moral, and material landscapes provided by the last chapter, this chapter looks more deeply at ideologies of language and translation in Chinese medicine. By ideologies of language, I am talking here about "any sets of beliefs about language articulated by the users as a rationalization or justification of perceived language structure and use" (Silverstein 1979: 193). I am talking, in other words, about what people in contemporary Chinese medicine think language *is* and how they understand what language *does* and *should do,* that is, how the use (or nonuse) of language is justified. By extension, when I speak of "ideologies of translation," I am referring to what people think translation is, what translation does, and what the structure of translation in Chinese medicine should be. All of the participants in the present study, from students, to teachers, to translators, have distinct, sometimes contradictory, and often shifting ideas about both language and translation. Such ideas, not surprisingly, are very much intertwined with each other, with ideologies of language often forming the basis of various ideologies of translation.

These divergent viewpoints are readable in the everyday ways people talk about Chinese medicine. They are also especially visible in the very heated international "translation debates," also referred to as the "nomenclature" or "terminology" debates. These debates are sometimes acrimonious conversations about language, terminology, and translation. They are carried out, in the West, on several popular Internet discussion groups, at formal conferences, in informal meetings among participants, and in several trade journals, including *American Acupuncturist* (Burke 2006; Ergil and Ergil 2006; Felt 2006a; Flaws 2006a; Given 2006; Rosenberg 2006; Shen 2006; Shima 2006), *Clinical Acupuncture and Oriental Medicine* (Beinfield and Korngold 2001; Wiseman 2001b), and *The Journal of Chinese Medicine* (Buck 2000; Felt 2000; Flaws 2000; Maciocia 2000; Wiseman 2000a). As language affects everybody, debate participation is not limited to authors and other scholars. Students, practitioners, and teachers also actively participate on a regular basis. Nor are such debates only occurring in the West. They have also received a great deal of attention from Chinese scholars and practitioners. Beginning in May 2003, for example, the well-known and widely circulated Chinese language *Journal of Chinese Integrative Medicine* (中西医结合学报 *Zhongxiyi Jiehe Xuebao)* started including a monthly section titled "Research on English Translation of TCM" (see Cao 2006; Li 2007, 2008a–f, 2009a, b, 2010; Li and Pan 2009a–c; Niu 2003, 2004, 2005, 2006; Yang 2007). In recent years, several other journals in China have followed suit, publishing regular articles on the translation of Chinese medicine. Another integrative medicine–themed journal, the *Chinese Journal of Integrated Medicine,* for example, has published several bilingual articles featuring debates between translators and scholars with diverse points of view, as well as overall perspectives on the debates themselves (Chen and Lu 2004; Hui and Pritzker 2007; Wiseman 2006; Xie 2002a, b, 2003b; Xie and White 2005).

The discussions, in both Western and Chinese debates, invariably revolve around several main issues, all of which are examined in more detail below. Briefly, there are struggles over whether Chinese medicine is best conveyed via a "source-oriented" or "target-oriented" method of translation, referring to the choices that translators make in either retaining the foreign nature of the material (source-oriented) or changing grammatical, terminological, and stylistic features of the text to make it more palatable in the receiving culture (target-oriented). Related to this, there is a great deal of debate over the use of biomedical terminology in the translation of Chinese medicine. There is also dispute about whether translation is ultimately possible across the great East-West linguistic divide. Finally, there is major disagreement over whether or not there should be a standardized terminology for the translation of Chinese medical texts, an issue that encompasses many smaller debates such as the technicality of Chinese medical language and the clinical and educational relevance of language in Chinese medicine.

Although often technical and related to specific terms, both the American and international debates, which often overlap (see Bruno 2008), also often generate extreme emotional expression. True to Gal's statement that "language ideologies are never only about language" (2005: 24), the language ideologies and ideologies of translation apparent in this complex field are deeply tied to notions of authenticity, personhood, and what Chinese medicine ultimately is. "This is the heart of the translation debate," writes one observer of the debates in an unpublished document that circulated through the community in 2001. "It is not about words, it is about what we believe Chinese medicine to be and how its literature can be rendered in English, learned, and taught." Such issues make the language debates in Chinese medicine a rich topic of study for anthropology, as struggles over translation involve multiple epistemologies of truth wherein different kinds of evidence, different ideas about what Chinese medicine is, and different notions of what language is, are used as valid bases for divergent ideologies of translation. In this chapter, I therefore view the ideologies about language and the translation debates themselves as "zones of encounter" in which Chinese medicine is continually made and remade through dialogues about language and translation. In other words, ideas about language (section one) and translation (section two) do more than theorize how translation should be done. From the perspective of living translation, such dialogues directly mediate, and often enact, translation.

Ideologies of Language

This section examines some of the major ideologies of language—notions of what language is, what it does, and how it should be structured or used—that exist in the diverse field of Chinese medicine as it is studied, taught, and practiced in translation. The ideologies explored here include the following: (1) language is arbitrary; (2) language determines thought/worldview; (3) language is a tool; and (4) language is cultural capital. These ideologies are not necessarily exclusive, nor are they inflexible. Like the moral landscape of Chinese medicine, ideologies of language in this field are multiple, and particular individuals can and often do subscribe to more than one at different times, even at the same time. As they provide the foundation for the ideologies of translation included in the next section, as well as they often mediate the enactment of translation itself, it is important to look here at each of these ideas about language separately, as ideal visions of what participants think language is and how it should be managed and structured in Chinese medicine.

Ideology: Language is Arbitrary

As highlighted in the last chapter, the contemporary Western emphasis on intuition, personal process, and spirituality in CAM generally and Chinese medicine specifically generates ambivalence about language, where experiences with spirit or deep Self are understood as prelinguistic and impossible to put in words. This came to light in several students' comments quoted above, as for example when Julia discusses the arbitrariness of translations for *qi*. "It is *qi*," she says. "Learn it." The idea is that *qi*, or any concept in Chinese medicine, transcends language barriers. Oren expresses this beautifully when he explains his perspective on language in Chinese medicine, "I think it's a universal medicine. Universal concepts. It could've been developed in any language, with any characters." The universality of "the medicine," also noted above, is rooted in the notion of Spirit, as expressed in the universal human body. Again, Julia: "You know, I mean, people who have never heard of *qi* before still have *qi;* it's not like you need a word for it in order for it to be a reality in your life, you know?" This sentiment is also commonly found in popular works, many of which cite the *Tao Te Ching (Dao De Jing),* quoted above. This ancient text thus states, "The way (*dao*) that can be spoken is not the constant [alt. translation: eternal] way." From the vantage point of universal, spiritual experience, this is often interpreted as a statement saying that language is simply an abstraction—from Spirit, from experience, from Truth. This perspective is not arbitrary. It arises from a moral framework of healing, spirituality, and self, a deeply felt personal reality that true healing is beyond language, described in depth in the last chapter.

It also, I want to emphasize here, reveals a set of distinctly Western ideologies of language. I am referring to longstanding notions that (a) language is merely referential to or designative of a separate reality, or of "things" in the world, and can therefore be listed in dictionaries (Bellos 2011; Silverstein 1979; Taylor 1985); (b) language is unimportant in comparison with a supposedly universal divine Truth, that it is merely an abstraction or even *dis*traction from that Truth (Bauman and Briggs 2003; Taylor 1985: 223); and (c) language is the mere "external clothing of thought" (Taylor 1985: 223).

The notion that language is referential of a separate reality "out there"—that *qi,* for example, is a "thing" regardless of the word—is common in contemporary Chinese medicine in the West. The origins of this common western idea can be traced, explains Bellos, to the Bible:

> And out of the ground the LORD God formed every beast of the field and every fowl of the air; and brought them unto Adam to see what he would call them: and whatsoever Adam called every living creature, that was the name thereof (Genesis 2:19 as cited in Bellos 2011: 85).

Bellos proposes that this biblical verse has shaped the way Westerners view language. "It says that language was, to begin with, and in principle still is, a list of words; and that words are the names of things (more particularly, the names of living things). Also, it says very succinctly that language is not among the things that God created but an arbitrary invention of humankind, sanctioned by divine assent" (Bellos 2011: 85). This idea that language is arbitrary and not in the realm of God creates what Bellos calls the "thingification" of language in Western thought. Dictionaries, as lists of words, compound this idea. "Dictionaries alone aren't responsible for the thingification of natural languages, but they crystallized a peculiar modern view of what it means to have a language" (Bellos 2011: 99). This ideology compels a distinct ambivalence toward language, a sense that it is arbitrary. For Western students of Chinese medicine, it initiates a turn toward the body and toward a felt experience of concepts that live in the universal realm of Spirit. It further indexes the ideology that language is unimportant in comparison with a supposedly universal divine Truth, that in this sense it is merely an abstraction or even *dis*traction from that Truth (Bauman and Briggs 2003; Taylor 1985: 223). This is also a deeply religious view of language, tied to the parable of Babel and the notion that, prior to the fall into differentiation, there was a language of "pure meaning" that was universal (Bellos 2011: 249). A related ideology of language that follows from this is that language is the mere "external clothing of thought" (Taylor 1985:223). Again, here there is a disdain for language as a "great seducer, tempting us to be satisfied with mere words, instead of focusing on the ideas they designate" (Taylor 1985: 225). The priority then becomes the *idea* of *qi*, the universal felt Truth of *qi*, rather than the word. As I have shown, this is not only an abstract "idea" about language, but a belief that has moral implications for the ways in which Chinese medicine is learned and practiced as an embodied, spiritual medicine that can be apprehended and put into practice without deep concern for precise words.

Ideology: Language Determines Thought/Worldview

There is another, very much related idea about language in Western conceptions of Chinese medicine. I am talking here about a popularized version of the theory of linguistic relativity. Also known as the "Sapir-Whorf hypothesis," this theory arises out of von Humboldt's thesis that "in each language only a part of the complete thought we have in mind is expressed" (Foley 1997: 195). In its strongest version of linguistic determinism, the people who speak a certain language are enclosed "in an invisible web of sounds and meanings, so that each nation is imprisoned by its language, a language further fragmented by historical eras, by social classes, by generations" (Paz 1992 [1971]: 154). It is important to note that the anthropologists often credited (and/or blamed) with developing linguistic relativity along cultural lines, Edward Sapir and Benjamin Lee Whorf, both acknowledged a dynamic interplay between culture, language, and individuals (Sapir 1958 [1932]; Whorf 1956 [1941]) and actually refuted the strong form of linguistic determinism. In anthropology, moreover, there has been a great deal of debate over the limits of such theories (Gumperz and Levinson 1996; Lucy 1992). In the popular imagination, however, the overall theory has often been interpreted as a blanket statement about the tendencies of all people who speak a given language to think in a certain way.

In Chinese medicine, the ideology of linguistic determinism and linguistic relativity shows up in students' ideas about language, especially notions of the incommensurability of Chinese, English, and other Western languages. Tricia, a French woman in her first quarter, thus talks about how difficult it is to understand the Chinese terms of Chinese medicine without having been brought up in the culture:

> I think that you must have been—you should have been born in China, brought up in China, completely immersed in that culture. 'Cause this is—this is *very* much, I think, culture, and *beliefs,* and having been able to read Chinese since you were a kid, and speak it, you know? In everyday life—I think at that point you might have a real understanding of—well, it's not even understanding. I think you don't understand it necessarily with your *head,* as you understand it with your *gut.* You understand it with your intuition. I think that's almost—that's why it's hard, because that intuition is based on, you know, (pause) the *culture* behind it. So it's just—between just French and English already you see a lot of you know, this—we're just going one word to another, or there're just subtleties obviously, you understand the *subtlety* … and just those characters [in Chinese medicine]—they're just poetic on their own. I mean, but you know, it's a different way of communicating and writing—it's just a different concept. It's a different nature.

For certain scholars and practitioners in Chinese medicine, the idea that it is a "different nature," as Tricia here calls it, holds a lot of ground. Indeed, in American Chinese medicine, "the East and West are discursively constructed as important philosophical bases from which to understand Chinese medicine" (Ho 2004: 70). The East, in this diametrical opposition "is presented as pluralistic and based on nature, *yin/yang,* notions of *qi,* energy, and balance … In contrast, the West is a way of thinking of the world that draws from biology, modern science and the scientific method, and a system based on physical evidence, standardization, and proof" (Ho 2004: 7). In some contemporary American Chinese medical circles, it has further led to the notion that Chinese is inherently better to think *holistically* with, because it is so different from English. Additionally, it leads to the view that, because of our different linguistic biases, *we* can see things in Chinese medicine that *they* cannot:

> It is natural to strive to understand the mind of Chinese medicine by comparing its linguistic and cultural constructs and metaphors with our own. While a Westerner may never grasp all of the nuances present in the source language of Chinese medicine, and thus never gain the breadth and depth of understanding of a native speaker on the other hand a Western thinker may see something in the ideas that the Chinese themselves would never discover precisely because of the limitations of their own language and culture (Beinfield and Korngold 2001: 154).

As Beinfield and Korngold here express, the notion that fundamental differences between an Eastern or Chinese and Western or American mindset leads quickly to the idea that we are both limited and privileged because of the differences and that determines the way we can apprehend the world. On top of this cultural difference, the ancientness of Chinese medical texts is seen as creating a divide between contemporary Western culture and the culture of ancient Chinese medicine (Bensky et al. 2006; Shen 2006; Shima 2006). In terms of the way participants view language, these fundamental dichotomies between East and West, past and present, rapidly translate into the notion that Chinese is so different from English that there is ultimately no way to bridge this divide in language.

The idea that Chinese is incommensurable with English (or French) creates tension for many of the students, as they are aware that the medicine they are studying originally came from China. The only way past this is to fall back on the idea of language being a distraction and to figure out how to get back to the universal. Thus Michael, in his second quarter, explains that because of the "big gap" between languages, he focuses instead on the "energy":

> Growing up in Greece, there are certain things that you cannot express in the English—or even if you express it, it doesn't make sense absolutely because the thinking part—you're not *wired* to think that particular way. It has to do with the culture a lot as well—so I think there will be always a big *gap*. And that's why I base myself, not on understanding the text, but rather when I study the Chinese medicine, but rather feel that *energy*, and go with the energy, because a human being is a human being, and, you know, once you're more aware of energies, then you'll be able to apply that more, you see.

Likewise, Sarah, toward the end of her first year, discusses the importance of getting to "the concept behind the character":

> When you have that cultural barrier, I think it's important but also difficult to get a well-rounded translation, definition. That doesn't just come from words. It comes from immersing yourself in that cultural mindset, and understanding that it's not just words, it's not just definitions. You have to feel out the whole concept behind the character.

Feeling the concept, getting behind the character, getting "under the hood" of the limits imposed by language, as it were, becomes the goal of students learning Chinese medicine in the United States. Again, "It is *qi*. Learn it." The priority remains the idea of *qi*, the universal felt Truth of *qi*, rather than the word.

Another obvious way to get past the cultural barrier posed by linguistic incommensurability is to learn Chinese. Generally speaking, however, acupuncturists and students in the United States "neither speak nor read Chinese and feel no need to do so" (Barnes 2003: 6). Many students and practitioners identify more with the search for an authentic practice in the context of their contemporary lives, rather than in a search for historical or linguistic accuracy. "These practitioners do not define themselves as scholars or historians," writes Barnes, "but as holders of a working knowledge that approximates aspects of the curriculum in Chinese medical schools" (2003: 6). The "working knowledge" Barnes here refers to is understood as a technical skill that utilizes secondary sources as providers of general instruction, but also relies heavily on self-referenced experience. For these students, the development of intuitive skills through listening to their teachers, their patients, and their deep selves, is sufficient. In the present study, for example, Michael explains why he has no interest in learning Chinese:

> I don't see the necessity of learning Chinese. You know, because energy, you know, is energy. And the way they may translate it in Chinese (.) you know, energy that you feel in your body. If you have awareness in your body, it doesn't matter where you are and what language you speak, you will feel the energy. You see?

For many students like Michael, translations may or may not be haphazard. It does not matter. *Qi* is *qi*. It is energy. Learn it.

Many students do recognize that learning Chinese is important, but the institutional support does not exist. As mentioned above, very few schools require any Chinese language training, and most of those that do offer only a one-quarter class in basic medical Chinese. For the students in the present study, there are tensions between institutional requirements and a developing sense of the value that learning Chinese would add to their clinical practice. In the school where I conducted my research, one quarter of Chinese medical language is required and can be taken at any time during the course of the four years of study. Because they are not particularly encouraged to take this class early, however, many students end up taking it when they are interns and have very little time to devote to language study.

Despite this conflict, some students do take the course, on their own initiative, in the early stages of their study. Even when students do learn some Chinese, however, both ideologies of language as arbitrary as well as ideologies of linguistic relativity are often reinforced. Oren, quoted above, took Chinese during his first quarter of school. He discusses how the class helped him to appreciate the "connection" between Chinese and English. He found it interesting, but for him, it further reinforced the arbitrariness of language:

> So I have an elementary understanding now of the direct relationship, the direct correspondence, between the characters and the concepts, which I find very helpful. At the same time, I guess it made me realize that it's still a language. It's still arbitrary. Some people think that the medicine couldn't have developed the way that it did without the Chinese language. I don't think that at all.

This is the context in which he offers his understanding of Chinese medicine as universal, but also complements it with a new appreciation for the beauty of Chinese, as a tool for "capturing" the universal ideas:

> It could've been developed in any language, with any characters. But I think the Chinese characters had a particular fluidity and capability of capturing the concepts in a way that English and other languages perhaps couldn't. So that illuminated that for me.

In studying Chinese, Oren thus accesses both the arbitrariness of language as well as experiencing a taste of the relativity of language in Chinese medicine. Sarah, who takes Chinese in her third quarter, has an even stronger experience. For her, learning Chinese underscores the incommensurability in the way of thinking and learning between Chinese and English:

> I feel like I'm understanding the Chinese terms differently, but I'm realizing there's so much more to understand that, you know, between our culture that learns linearly, that learns word for word what everything is supposed to mean, versus looking at a symbol and understanding it conceptually, understanding how it has morphed into what it is in modern-day Chinese. I think it doesn't give me a better understanding of the Chinese words and the concepts. It gives me a better idea of the fact of how much I *don't* know, how much more I *do* want to understand, and the fact that if we are going to have any sort of idea what these concepts mean in their true Chinese sense, I have a lot more studying to do, I have a lot more characters to learn. And it's only scratching the surface; it's only scratching the very, very surface.

This was humbling for Sarah. For both Oren and her, it opened their eyes to a new way of appreciating the language of Chinese medicine and yet at the same time underscored the incommensurability and arbitrariness of language.

Ideology: Language Is a Tool

For some teachers, authors, and translators, the lack of Chinese language in U.S. Chinese medical programs is simply unacceptable. As Bob Flaws, a translator and author of a multitude of English-language Chinese medical texts, puts it, "What we believe is that in order to understand how to do Chinese medicine technically, you have to understand the words" (Emad 2006: 414). Flaws's position here highlights the technical reasons to learn Chinese, suggesting that it simply makes you a better practitioner. But Flaws and others have also repeatedly emphasized that learning Chinese is important simply to have access to the vast library of texts in Chinese, in other words, to *listen* directly to the authors of Chinese texts. In these arguments, there is a distinct ideology of language as a *tool* that also has a rich history in Western thought (Taylor 1985).

Several of the students in the present study who did choose to study Chinese also expressed versions of this ideology. After one quarter of medical Chinese, Julia further talked about feeling "empowered" by the idea that she could pick up a dictionary and begin to understand some of the Chinese texts after only one quarter:

> Just learning little sentences, you can start to see that it is possible that you could learn this? And so that in and of itself is really encouraging ... I mean, we translated the first paragraph of the *Huangdi Neijing,* and it was cool. It was like YEAH, you know, like looked it up in the little dictionary, and made it all happen. You know, I have my little dictionary now. Like I could, you know, I could—it would take me days and days, but I could—if I had to translate a medical text, I could do it. You know, maybe. ((laughs)) ... I totally feel empowered to do it. I don't feel like I don't have the tools to do it, you know what I mean, I know I could, like, access something if I really wanted to. And that feels really great, and so I really like that.

Julia's empowerment here derives from the fact that she feels that she has the tools to access Chinese texts, if she really wanted to. The ideology of language as tool starts to complement her previous understandings. Here, it is a tool for access, as described above, but interestingly, it is also a tool of empowerment that shows up in other ways. For example, both Julia and Treavor report feeling empowered, after learning a little bit of Chinese, to critique their non-Chinese-speaking instructors. After Julia begins to learn Chinese, for instance, she is bothered by the fact that none of her non-Chinese-speaking instructors pronounce the tones when they teach the Chinese words. Likewise, Treavor grows wary of many of the character etiologies offered by his non-Chinese-speaking instructors, often taking such explanations back to his Chinese books to confirm their inaccuracy.

Interestingly, language is also understood as a tool in the traditional Chinese ideology of language as an instrument for "deciphering classics to follow the example of former rulers" (Wang 1981; as cited in Hui 2009:158). In classical Chinese, this particular understanding of language led to the development of early dictionaries organized not by word lists but by associative semantics that offered a "tool for cultivating knowledge of more ancient texts" (Bellos 2011: 96). In this formulation, language, while not itself the eternal way or *dao,* is understood as part of the vast network that points back to it and is a window into it rather than an abstraction from it. Although Western teachers and students in the current study did not share this ideology of language, remnants of the core idea can be observed in some of the Chinese teachers' responses to questions about the meaning of specific terms. In chapter 4, for example, Dr. Liu, a teacher from mainland China working at the school where I conducted my research, responds to a student's inquiry about the meaning of the term *yin*, translated as "rheum," by drawing upon associated Chinese terms to index the network of concepts that relates back to classic Chinese texts. This strategy puts him in conflict with the type of meaning that the students are searching for and causes a disruption of the class that I explore in detail as a moment when translation is being enacted in interaction.

Ideology: Language as Cultural Capital

There is also an awareness among participants in the present study that language exists as a form of cultural capital. Bourdieu (1991) discusses the role of official state-mandated language forms in both constituting and regulating the linguistic market such that speakers of alternative linguistic forms must wage a constant battle to gain acceptance. Bourdieu, along with other scholars, approaches such linguistic forms as systems of cultural capital that function to regulate the position of speakers in the market (Bourdieu 1991; Irvine 1989; Woolard 1985). In Chinese medicine, the linguistic market is not only diverse, but it is, as of the present, quite unregulated by any official body. This gives rise to multiple ways of speaking—and of translating—Chinese medical terms. The power dynamics involved with the many different approaches to translating in this field, including ideologies for and against standardization, are discussed in detail below. Here, I want to focus more on the basic ideology of language as a form of cultural capital, a form of social qualification that has the power to both permit and constrain political, economic, and social mobility.

From this vantage point, participants in the translation of Chinese medicine into language and practice in the West have varying degrees of concern about the role of language in their social positioning. Many translators in both China and the West feel that the use of traditional, esoteric terms for the expression of Chinese medical concepts in English, for example, perpetuates the social positioning of Chinese medicine as an ancient form of healthcare, irrelevant to the progress of modern global medicine. They prefer biomedical terminology when speaking of Chinese medicine in English (Kendall 2002; Lei 2004; Niu 2003, 2004). Others feel strongly that the cultural heritage of Chinese medicine must be respected in language that reflects the historical context of its use. Viewing the language that is used to convey Chinese medicine in English as a form of cultural capital that positions the speakers in relation to the originators of the medicine, they argue for more traditional translations. For the students who are learning Chinese medicine and beginning to think about how they will use language to practice once they are licensed, there is also an awareness of how the linguistic forms that they choose will function as a form of social and cultural capital in the context of their own work. Oren, for example, professes a strong sense of distaste for the use of Chinese words at all in the English expression of Chinese medicine, arguing that it takes away his own authority as an expert:

> I think *yin* and *yang* should have their own English words. I don't think we should be running around using *pinyin*. Because that gives the Chinese an authority. This is the—English is the language that I'll be using in this culture, and if there are Chinese words thrown in here and there for the most important concepts? Then Chinese people will always have the authority.

Here, Oren directly links language to cultural authority, claiming that because he will be speaking English with his clients in this country, he should not be using any Chinese words. The use of Chinese words grants an authority to "Chinese people" that Oren would rather not accept in his own practice. The ideology of language as cultural capital is functioning here to structure Oren's choice of ways of speaking about Chinese medicine.

Section Discussion

In this section, I have shown that various ideologies of what language is and what it does permeate the learning of Chinese medicine in the contemporary United States.

Notions of language as arbitrary relate to the moral field surrounding Chinese medicine as a form of CAM in the United States. At the same time, such ideas are deeply tied to traditional Western ways of understanding language as referential and therefore arbitrary relative to spiritual Truth. Notions of linguistic relativity similarly reflect a long discourse about language and culture in Western thought, as well as work alongside moral ideologies of sameness and difference in Chinese medicine. Likewise for ideologies of language as a tool and language as cultural capital: these are deeply moral ideologies that come up more or less frequently in Chinese medicine and greatly impact the way it is interpreted, and used, in everyday practice. Such ideas about language also form the foundation for different ideologies of translation, examined in the next section.

Ideologies of Translation

Translation, perhaps not surprisingly, comes up quite often in the context of debates over what language is and how much language one should learn to access or grasp the meaning of Chinese medical concepts. The direct link is discussed quite explicitly in the international debates about translation and terminology in Chinese medicine, introduced above. This section draws upon statements made publicly in those debates—in print and at conferences—to get a better sense of some of participants' ideas about what translation in Chinese medicine is, what it does, and what it *should* do. As above, I separate the section into subsections based on different ideologies, including the following: (1) translation is bearing across or bringing over; (2) translation is a tool of power; (3) ideologies of the im/possibility of translation; and (4) ideologies of standardization in translation. These are all complex ideologies, and like ideologies of language, they are not necessarily mutually exclusive. Together, they constitute the terrain of talk about translation in Chinese medicine, rather than inflexible positions that specific individuals always espouse. Like ideologies of language and moral frameworks, it is thus perhaps useful to think of translation ideologies as available perspectives existing together in a landscape of possibility that, as a whole, plays a mediating role in the enactment of translation in Chinese medicine.

Ideology: Translation is Bearing Across or Bringing Over

The idea that translation is "bearing across" or "bringing over" is a common understanding in Western thought as well as in Chinese medicine. This definition may seem obvious, as the etiology of the word "translation" actually expresses this very idea. "Translation," writes Bellos, "comes from two Latin words, *trans,* meaning 'across,' and the past form *latum* of the verb *ferre,* 'to bear.' The result of the word history is to give *translate* the meaning of 'bear across' or 'bring over'" (2011: 28). In this formulation, it follows that there are two opposing or different 'sides' that need to be somehow reconciled so that one side, the *source,* can be born across or brought over to the other, the *target.* In Chinese medicine, the source is China, and the source language is Chinese. The target, at least in the present volume, is the United States, and the target language is English. This may seem straightforward enough, as the following statement from Nigel Wiseman, a prominent and controversial translator in the field of Chinese medicine, clearly describes:

> Whether you are an educator planning curricula, a teacher planning a course, or a student or practitioner browsing in a bookshop, you should remember that whatever you know about Chinese medicine—I mean East Asian medicine as opposed to any Western rewrite of it—reaches you by the medium of translation. However many hands any item of knowledge passes through before it reaches you, it has, at one point or another, had to be translated into English (Wiseman 2000d: 6).

The idea here, again, is straightforward. Information originating in Chinese needs to be "brought over" into English for Westerners to use it. As I will discuss in detail in chapter 4, the awareness of this transfer permeates everyday interaction in the school where I conducted my ethnographic research. It is one way of imagining translation that almost everyone in the field agrees upon.

Before discussing some of the other ways in which translation is understood in Chinese medicine, it is important to consider several derivative ideas linked to the notion of translation as transfer. These are arguments or ways of conceptualizing translation that pertain in most Western dialogues about translation in general, and they also show up in conversations about the translation of Chinese medicine. First, when translation is conceptualized as 'bringing over,' then there must be some *thing* to be brought over. This something is usually conceptualized as "meaning":

> We do say *translate,* and we do think *transfer,* and because we think *transfer,* we have to find the complement or object of that verb. And in the mainstream tradition of Western thought about language, only one candidate has ever been thought suitable for the role: *meaning* (Bellos 2011: 33, italics in original).

This idea, that there is a thing—meaning—that must be carried across is deeply tied to the ideology of language as referential, as having an object out in the world, explained above. To continue with the example of *qi,* the meaning of the word must be conveyed, or carried over, from Chinese into English. This is not an easy task, and there are many ways to think about how to accomplish this in language as well as in the body.

Focusing on linguistic translation points us toward a second notion that emerges when translation is envisioned as transfer. It is the idea of *movement.* If translation is the carrying across of meaning, then the translator's task becomes to move such meaning across languages and cultures. Here, it is not only meaning that is conceptualized as being able to move, however. It is also the author, or the reader, that can be moved. From this perspective, a translator has two options: "Either the translator leaves the writer alone as much as possible and moves the reader toward the writer, or leaves the reader alone as much as possible and moves the writer toward the reader" (Schliermacher 1992 [1813]: 42). The image here is clear: there are two sides that exist apart from one another in time/space, and some sort of movement has to occur for communication to take place. Thus arise the notions of *source-oriented* and *target-oriented* translation. In a source-oriented approach, "one is concerned that the message in the receptor language should match as closely as possible the different elements in the source language" (Nida 2000 [1964]: 129). This kind of translation, Nida explains, "is designed to permit the reader to identify himself as fully as possible with a person in the source-language context, and to understand as much as he can of the customs, manner of thought, and means of expression" (2000 [1964]: 129). In Schliermacher's metaphor, the source-oriented approach moves the reader more toward the source, toward the meaning. A target-oriented translation, however, is not very much concerned with making the target reader move at all beyond his or her comfort zone, instead asking the writer to move toward the reader in translation. This is done by presenting the text as if it were originally written in the target language, making it unnecessary for the reader to understand much of the cultural context of the source text. The sociocultural implications of each choice have been discussed ad nauseam throughout history, and they are still very relevant today. In Chinese medicine, this debate is equally long-lived and will be discussed in detail below.

A third conceptualization that arises from the ideology of translation-as-transfer is the notion of the existence of a language barrier. "Would we have ever thought up the idea of a 'language barrier' if our word for translator did not imply something like 'truck driver'?" asks Bellos (2011: 33). Although I question the sole responsibility of the word "translation" for the development of the idea of a language barrier, it is worth pointing out here that the metaphorical entailments of ideologies of "translation as transfer of meaning"—as well as the metaphor itself—are deeply bound up in the idea of languages as representative of vastly different worldviews that somehow need to be moved toward one another in the process of translation. In this sense, it is deeply intertwined with the ideology of linguistic relativity and even determinism, in which barriers are seen to exist between languages. In Chinese medicine, as in other fields, the answer to the question of whether such barriers are penetrable at all can be found in further ideologies of the possibility and the impossibility of translation, also discussed below.

I want to close this section with a word of caution about the apparent obviousness of the ideology of translation as transfer. It is not the only way to think about translation. Bellos, for example, makes it clear that "there are lots of other metaphors available in many languages, including our own, and they have just as much right to our attention as the far from solid conceit of the ferry operator or trucker who carries something from A to B" (2011: 29). Bellos explains that translation was conceptualized as "turning" in ancient Sumerian and Latin (2011: 29). In Chinese, the term for translation 译 *yi*, has been understood over time as "those who transmit the words of the tribes in the four directions; to state in an orderly manner and be conversant in the words of the country and those outside the country; to exchange, that is to say, to change and replace the word of one language by another to achieve mutual understanding; to exchange, that is to say, to take what one has in exchange for what one does not have" (2011: 32–33). Although there are similarities, none of these ways of conceptualizing translation involve the notion of translation as transfer or bearing across. By sharing metaphors of turning, transmitting, and exchanging, Bellos thus demonstrates that the idea of bearing across some kind of divide is not necessarily critical for understanding translation. In the field of translation studies, this core metaphor of translation-as-transfer is currently being reexamined and deeply questioned as more dialogic theories of translation emerge. Such dialogic models of translation emphasize the mutual exchange that occurs in translation and highlight translation as an ongoing process. These models, in fact, form the foundation of living translation as described in this book. In this chapter, however, I would like to focus on what kinds of ideas people in Chinese medicine have about translation and how these ideas themselves mediate the overall process of living translation, the enactment of translation on a broad scale.

Ideologies: Translation is Im/possible

Notions of source-oriented and target-oriented translation, and the underlying notion of translation as bearing across, have given rise to the age-old debate about whether translation is possible or not (see Anelo 2005; Bellos 2011; Darnell 2000; Liu 1995, 1999; Malinowski 1978; Ortega y Gasset 1937 [1992]). The notion that translation is impossible, for example, derives quite naturally from both ideologies of language as referential and language as determinative of thought. If language describes things, Bellos explains, "then translation would clearly be impossible for almost everything we say except for our fairly infrequent references to a very large range of specific material things" (2011: 84). Likewise, if languages are accepted as determining the way we think, then creating a similar thought pattern by means of using another language is only something one can approximate or attempt. It is not truly possible. On the other hand, the possibility of translation emerges in arguments that see language as capable of talking about "anything that comes up" (2011: 89). In other words, if the possibility of understanding different perspectives and different contexts is inherent in language, then translation is possible, whether or not one subscribes to the ideology of linguistic relativity. In what Anelo (2005) calls "universal rationalism," moreover, translation is possible because of the universal foundation for language in shared biological and psychological realities. Translators, and commenters on translation, have endlessly discussed the implications and ramifications of each ideological pole—from translation is impossible to translation is possible. They usually agree on an ideal falling somewhere between the two.

In Chinese medicine, the discussion of the im/possibility of translation can be quite heated. There are many who feel that completely accurate translation in this vast field, especially because of the fundamental linguistic divide between East and West, past and present, is ultimately impossible (Beinfield and Korngold 2001; Bensky et al. 2006; Deadman 2000; Fratkin 2006; Shen 2006; Shima 2006). Giovanni Maciocia, a well-known and well-regarded author of several major English-language textbooks in Chinese medicine, thus argues that there is simply no one-to-one correlation between Chinese and English words:

> I personally feel that it is simply impossible to translate Chinese medicine terms into a Western language. The best we can achieve is an approximation of meaning. Most Chinese medicine terms have more than one meaning and therefore any translation that focuses on one meaning only is necessarily an approximation. Thus, by definition, there is no "correct" translation of Chinese medicine terms (Maciocia 2000: 50).

The "approximation of meaning" that Maciocia here refers to often draws not only upon a single, dominant Chinese meaning, but also upon the meaning that makes the most sense to Western readers. Alterations are thus bound to occur and should in fact be welcomed as American authors adjust Chinese medicine to make it more familiar and useful for their English-speaking, Western audiences. These alterations are, moreover, not seen as aberrations but as necessary and innocent moves to translate the material into a different cultural context. For Maciocia and other scholars who see translation as impossible, then, a target-oriented translation approach is decidedly better, as it allows for the "*acceptance* and *use* of Chinese medicine in the West" through "culturally accessible" renditions that make no claim to be translations and do not aim to transmit "*authentic* Chinese traditional medical knowledge" (Beinfield and Korngold 2001: 150, italics in original).

In opposition to this view of incommensurability, and despite the differences that exist between Chinese and Western cultures and languages, others insist that it is still possible to translate Chinese medical material using a source-oriented approach. Nigel Wiseman thus states that, although it might not be possible to translate "every idea and nuance of meaning" (Wiseman 2000b: 4), source-oriented translation is still very much a possibility. Unschuld agrees, arguing that part of what makes this possible is the existence of what he called "generic terms" that "remain identical through the centuries and millennia" (1989: 101). He points to the term "blood" for example, saying that although "the conceptual associations … may vary significantly in the course of time" (Unschuld 1989: 101), the basic material reality of it does not differ in time or place. Wiseman, in concert with Paul Zmiewski, further writes that striving to find English equivalents that capture more than one of the multiple meanings of Chinese terms is another strategy for responsibly achieving source-oriented translation (Wiseman and Zmiewski 1989).

Ideology: Translation is a Tool of Power

Most discussions of translation, including especially notions of translation-as-transfer, lead immediately to politics, power, and control. Schliermacher, for example, points out that a target-oriented translation is "strictly speaking, not … translation" (1992 [1813]: 53). Instead, he notes that this type of translation is an "imitation" or rendition, one that inevitably leads to a fundamental transformation of the message as it is rendered in the target language. Although some scholars believe that this transformation is necessary and natural, and happens at both intentional and unintentional levels (Reiss 2000 [1971]), others have noted that the choice between a source-oriented or target-oriented orientation is the critical juncture at which translation moves beyond being only a linguistic activity and becomes a sociocultural and political practice embedded in complex relations of power. Citing the Romans as an example, Nietzsche thus demonstrates how imperialism works through target-oriented translation:

> And then Roman antiquity itself: how violently, and at the same time how naively, it pressed its hand upon everything good and sublime in the older periods of ancient Greece! Consider how the Romans translated this material to suit their own age and how intentionally as well as heedlessly they wiped away the wing-dust of the butterfly moment! … They [the poets] seemed to ask us: 'Should we not make antiquity to suit our own purposes and make *ourselves* comfortable in it? … In those days, indeed, to translate meant to conquer … And all this was done with the very best conscience as a member of the Roman empire, without realizing that such actions constituted theft (Nietzsche 1992 [1882]: 69).

Nietzsche here highlights the role of translation in the Roman imperialist mission to conquer foreign lands, showing how a target-oriented approach to translation exposes an ethnocentric mindset that literally steals from other cultures. Friedrich further explains this process, revealing how, in the Latin imperialist quest, "translation meant transformation in order to mold the foreign into the linguistic structures of one's own culture" (1992 [1965]: 12). As Venuti points out, this type of "translational imperialism" is no less of an issue today, when target-oriented translation liberally changes the source text to submit to the expectations of the target culture. "Translating," he explains, "is always ideological because it releases a domestic remainder, an inscription of values, beliefs, and representations linked to historical moments and social positions in the domestic culture" (Venuti 2000: 485). From this perspective, the translator is imbued with the unique power of transformation as enacted through language.

The role of power in translation raises issues of faithfulness and morality that urge Nietzsche, Friedrich, and Venuti, among others, to argue strongly for the legitimacy of a source-oriented over a target-oriented approach. "The lion's share of the literature on translation and interpretation," writes Wadensjö, "topicalizes this issue as a fundamentally *moral* one, a question of how to remain faithful to original speakers and/or stay loyal to professional norms" (1998: 30). From this perspective, the task of the translator is couched in a moral obligation to the one whom he or she is translating.

In Chinese medicine, the greatest champion of a source-oriented approach incorporating cultural context is Nigel Wiseman. Wiseman terminology, sometimes known as "Wisemanese," is based on the source-oriented method of Chinese medical translation he developed in his doctoral thesis titled "Translation of Chinese Medical Terminology: A Source-Oriented Approach" (Wiseman 2000c). His translation philosophy is based on the belief that "to transmit Chinese medical knowledge to the West, we must translate, not reinvent" (Wiseman 2002b: 22). A source-oriented approach, he argues, is therefore necessary.

Relating the need for a source-oriented approach to the esteem in which the translator holds the target language and culture, Wiseman further argues that a source-oriented approach is the only proper way in which to appropriately respect genuine Chinese medical wisdom. Basing his analysis firmly upon scholars in translation studies who advocate a source-oriented approach for sociocultural reasons, Wiseman contends that the widespread tendency for Westerners to rely on a target-oriented style of translation for Chinese medical texts reflects an ethnocentric and colonialist mentality. "Things would almost certainly have been otherwise," he asserts, "had the West been under Chinese domination for centuries, and educated Westerners could all speak and write Chinese fluently" (Wiseman 2000b: 7). Wiseman thus adopts Venuti's style of "abusive fidelity" (Venuti 1992) by using obscure English terms to translate the essence of ancient Chinese medical meanings. According to both Venuti and Wiseman, the obscurity or unfamiliarity of the terms requires readers to stretch their minds to grasp the full meaning of a given term. As such, Wiseman sees himself as working within a morally grounded source-oriented framework in which he moves the reader more toward the writer and not vice versa.

When a source-oriented approach to translation is not used, Wiseman, along with several others, argues that it leads to fundamental distortions of Chinese medical knowledge. These distortions often relate directly to the ideologies that draw people to the medicine in the first place. For example, both Wiseman and Unschuld suggest that the tendency for Westerners to view Chinese medicine through the lens of "alternative healthcare ideologies" that see Chinese medicine as inherently more natural, holistic, and person-centered than biomedicine leads to many inaccuracies in linguistic representation (Unschuld 2003; Wiseman 2001a). They see the tendency for selective and incomplete translation, for example, as especially problematic:

> In Chinese medicine, metaphors of killing, defense and attack have been taken for granted since ancient times. This figurative use of language, however, does not appear in the version of Chinese medicine propagated in the West ... In contrast to reports from the battlefield of modern immunology, the theory of TCM freed of its martial metaphors gives the impression that it can lead patients back to the harmony of the great whole. It offers solace where modern medicine offers only the uncertainty of a murderous battle (Unschuld 2003: 218–219).

In this case, Unschuld argues, the obfuscation of certain aspects of Chinese medicine (metaphors of killing, defense, and attack) serves to create an impression that Chinese medicine is a completely gentle form of care that only uses natural metaphors. This works to position Chinese medicine as biomedicine's gentle opposite, when in many cases it is not. This not only distorts the historical truth, but potentially limits the therapeutic effect of Chinese medical approaches that can effectively "attack" certain pernicious influences.

Another instance where this type of betrayal tends to occur, argues Wiseman, is in the inaccurate portrayal of the traditional importance of scholarship in Chinese medicine, where physicians were expected to be learned scholars as well, to memorize and think deeply about the classic texts. By simply linking it to other forms of alternative medicine, Chinese medical authors in the United States too often promote the dichotomy often posited between "book-learning" and "experience" or "intuition":

> Chinese medicine is identified as an alternative medicine and, as such, is assumed to possess the characteristics that all alternative medicines are assumed to possess. Among those characteristics are an emphasis on the value of the clinical encounter rather than on "book learning." This characterization is completely erroneous from two points of view. First, in the tradition of Chinese medicine that Westerners are trying to adopt, book learning is very important. Chinese students were expected to study the classics in detail and even to memorize them. Second, this book knowledge is not all theoretical. Most of the literature of Chinese medicine is much more closely related to clinical practice than the theoretical knowledge of Western medicine (Wiseman 2002b: 19).

The cultivation of strong clinical skills in Chinese medicine, Wiseman contends, requires both text-based study as well as clinical experience and intuitive development. From the perspective of the alternative medicine community of Chinese medicine in the United States, however, Wiseman argues that the disdain for language, the preference "to think of Chinese medical healing [as resting upon] on sublime knowledge that transcends the normal plane of human experience which can be communicated in words" (2002b: 19) sets the stage for the lack of regard for precise terminology in translation. If Chinese medicine is a purely intuitive, holistic medicine learned by practice, then it follows that there is no need to bother getting the language right. Wiseman argues that such a perspective is based on an ethnocentric and deeply immoral disregard of the source culture.

A colonialist mentality, Wiseman thus claims, is responsible for the target-oriented ideology of translation that denies the Chinese sources the respect they deserve and twists them into the Western narrative of alternative healthcare. This bias, Unschuld also argues, effectively excludes Chinese authors from the Western market:

> Among the bestselling books on Chinese medicine in the English-speaking world, not a single title has been authored by a Chinese author. Chinese authors are unfamiliar with the fears and expectations of Western audiences. Hence they do not find the right words to be accepted by those in the West who are interested in the conceptual message behind the practice of TCM and acupuncture (Unschuld 2003: 221).

A factor that makes this representation even more problematic, Wiseman argues, is the fact that many of the supposedly translated sources of Chinese medicine "do not contain any explicit statement to the effect that they were translated or compiled from primary Chinese or other primary Oriental sources (Japanese, Korean) and their bibliographies suggest that no primary sources were consulted in their compilation" (Wiseman 2000c: 200). Wiseman thus claims that with this erasure of primary sources, Westerners thereby steal the power of representation away from the source culture.

This is not the only way in which translation in Chinese medicine is conceptualized as a tool of power. A prominent translator in China, Xie Zhufan, has written extensively about the ways in which translations that "foreignize" Chinese medicine through the use of traditional terminology actually perpetuate the inferiority of Chinese medicine vis-à-vis modern biomedicine. Both in his book, *On the Standard Nomenclature of Traditional Chinese Medicine*, and in a series of articles in *China Journal of Integrated Medicine*, Xie articulates his motivations for choosing biomedically oriented terms to translate Chinese medicine, arguing that English terminology for the translation of Chinese medical material should be based on modern biomedical (Western medical) concepts so as to accurately represent Chinese medicine as a viable medical system appropriate for use in international contexts (Xie 2002a, b, 2003a, b; Xie and White 2005, 2006). Translations that rely upon biomedical terms, he maintains, also effectively bring Chinese medicine into the current age, saving it from being considered a cultural relic in the modern world:

> In short, the proper use of Western medical terms is necessary and may facilitate the correct understanding of TCM. Insisting on intentionally keeping TCM terminology apart from Western medical terms in every aspect will make a false impression that TCM is an esoteric system of medicine (Xie 2003a: 24).

Xie thus asserts that not only does the use of biomedical terms to represent Chinese medical concepts serve the project of bringing Chinese medicine into the current age, but it also helps in making Chinese medicine feel more familiar and accessible to Western audiences.

This familiarity, Xie further contends, facilitates a bridging of the gap between the two systems, which is ultimately feasible because most medical terms and concepts "are not usually culture-specific" (2003a: 10). "Except for some metaphorical expressions," he continues, "for most of these terms English equivalents can be found," going on to suggest that the terminology used in the International Classification of Diseases (ICD) should be taken as the standard for translating Chinese medicine (2003a: 10). Xie thus bypasses any issues relating to supposed cultural difference, claiming that Chinese medical translation should proceed from a scientific basis rather than a literary one. Literary translation, he argues, which is needed only for the translation of ancient poetry and literature, might require taking ancient cultural factors into consideration, but not so in medicine, where "the ancient cultural background, which exerted an impact on the development of Chinese medicine … no longer plays an important role in the present practice of Chinese medicine" (2003a: 8). Wiseman and other Westerners' tendency to use traditional terminology to translate is therefore entirely unnecessary from Xie's vantage point. Not only does it obscure the medicine, making it seem like an antique instead of a legitimate science, it also puts too much weight on the need to appreciate ancient concepts to understand contemporary Chinese medical terms. A target-oriented translation prioritizing biomedicine is therefore more appropriate from Xie's point of view.

Xie Zhufan and Nigel Wiseman are not the only participants in the field of Chinese medical translation, of course, but their disparate views highlight the complex issues of power involved in discussions about source-oriented and target-oriented translation. Both share the ideology that translation is a tool of power, and yet they approach the discussion from vastly different understanding of power and different understandings of what constitutes the source of translation. The fact that they have engaged very publicly in conversations with each other about translation further invites an anthropological understanding of the way definitions of power articulate with ideologies of language and translation. In a series of articles, for example, Wiseman adamantly argues that Xie's preference for biomedical terminology is misguided, that the use of biomedical terms to translate Chinese medicine "destroys the integrity and independence of Chinese medical concepts" (Wiseman 2006: 225). From his perspective, biomedical terms linguistically map the biomedical body onto the traditional body of Chinese medicine, thereby negating it (Wiseman 2000c: 29). The basis of Xie's erroneous views, Wiseman claims, is his misunderstanding about who exactly Chinese medical material is being translated for:

> A fundamental reason why Professor Xie and his colleagues believe Western medical terms are appropriate is their belief that the main Western audience for Chinese medicine is the Western medical community. This is simply not true … According to one report, as few as 10 percent of practitioners of acupuncture are MDs; the rest are non-MDs … People who seriously study Chinese medicine are quite happy to learn terms for traditional Chinese medical concepts. Because they like Chinese medicine, they like to know the Chinese-style names (Wiseman 2006: 226–227).

Wiseman here refers to the audience for most Chinese medical texts in the United States, the students and practitioners who have turned to Chinese medicine as an alternative to biomedicine. Although as we saw above, he claims elsewhere that the desire for an alternative to biomedicine often misleads this population into misinterpretations of Chinese medicine, he argues here on their behalf, explaining that they actually do want to know the "real" Chinese medicine, the medicine that evolved over thousands of years of Chinese culture. For Wiseman, again, the real issue is cultural. Underlying his argument is a fundamental distinction between Chinese and biomedicine. As we have witnessed in his source-oriented approach to translation, to know the real Chinese medicine requires a concomitant cultural and linguistic knowledge. Xie's reasoning in regards to this issue, Wiseman claims, is skewed based on "a deep-seated sense of inferiority about Chinese medicine" (Wiseman 2006: 225) derived from the past century of having to scientize Chinese medicine:

> It is further interesting to note that the Chinese translators … on the whole favor a greater degree of Westernization than the Western translators … I suggest this is because, given the current wider intercultural state of affairs, Chinese people feel a far greater need to justify Chinese medicine in terms of modern medicine than Westerners do (Wiseman 2000c: 226).

Wiseman here deals a heavy blow to the very basis of Xie's understanding, alleging that his motivation to "biomedicize" Chinese medicine is based in cultural inferiority and "destroys the integrity and independence of Chinese medical concepts; it devalues Chinese medicine" (2006: 225). In linking Xie's target-oriented translation approach to the sociopolitical environment in which Chinese medicine was forced to accommodate to the broader trends toward Westernization and scientization that took over in China since the turn of the century, Wiseman thus positions himself as a cultural protector, defending authentic Chinese medicine when the Chinese themselves would have it otherwise. The irony of this position is not lost on Wiseman. It is a "pity," he writes, that Westerners are the ones who have to mine the classics to develop a source-oriented approach, "because Chinese participation would greatly benefit the transmission process and, indeed, would accord China its rightful position of international authority in its own medicine" (Wiseman 2001a: 49).

In the context of U.S. and international efforts to transmit Chinese medical information, all of this creates a messy debate over who has the cultural "rights" to translate the medicine into English. In calling Chinese medicine China's "own" medicine, for example, Wiseman professes that China rightly possesses the knowledge. In one sense, this ideologically privileges the Chinese to represent the material. Indeed, Wiseman writes elsewhere that "[i]f we acknowledge the Chinese as the originators of Chinese medicine, we must also acknowledge that they have a clear understanding of what is and is not a useful concept" (Wiseman 2000a: 46). In the case of biomedical terminology, however, he argues that the Chinese have, in effect, given up this right by "selling out" to imperialist expectations of scientific rigor. The notion of ownership, however, is also drawn upon by Xie and his supporters. Chen and Lu thus write that "[a]s ones who understand TCM with native language at the birthplace of TCM, we should take the responsibility for the formulation of the standard [English] nomenclature" (Chen and Lu 2004: 70). Both sides of this debate therefore profess a similar notion of origin and ownership to argue for different strategies of translation. The common denominator is the notion of translation as a tool of power, that by doing translation, one is enacting some form of power.

Ideologies: Translated Terminology Should/Should Not Be Standardized

In linguistic anthropology, standardization of language is a complex political issue. Lack of attention to variation, Woolard (1998) asserts, neglects the realities of working-class and minority community practices. Bauman and Briggs explain:

> The ideology of a monoglot and monologic standard has provided a charter not only for homogenizing national policies of language standardization and the regulation of public discourse, but also for theoretical frameworks that normalize and often essentialize one society-one culture one-language conceptions of the relationships among language, culture, and society (2000: 202).

Furthermore, the issue of a standardized, "proper" language is commonly associated with power, authority, and dominance in studies of language ideology (Bourdieu 1991; Gal 1989; Woolard 1998). It is for these reasons that Bourdieu suggests that the argument of "functionality" does not justify the institution of a standard form for language.

Standardized language, from this perspective, is a measure of control, of power, that is instituted primarily in schools (Bourdieu 1991). For these reasons, resistance to the standard are often the norm, enacted "when devalued linguistic strategies and genres are practiced despite denigration, and when these devalued practices propose or embody alternate models of the social world" (Gal 1989: 349). The struggle that is thus waged between ideologies captures a reality that standardized, rationalist models of language ignore. A similar perspective is taken by Herzfield in regard to translation: "The use of standardized translations … obliterates the play of actors' perhaps quite divergent intentions in favor of structural unity and images of social stability and equilibrium" (Herzfeld 2003: 115). The notion that any language, translated or otherwise, can be standardized suggests dominance and disregard for linguistic variation.

In Chinese medicine, there are fierce debates over the creation and imposition of a set of standardized terms for the translation of medical texts. As in linguistic anthropology, themes of dominance, resistance, and cultural/linguistic hegemony play a role in all sides of this debate. It is not cut and dried, however. In Chinese medicine, forces of power and authority are not clearly delineated, as in, for example, cases of government-mandated policy on language. This is due to the fact that, although different organizations from the World Health Organization (WHO) to the World Federation of Chinese Medical Societies (WFCMS) to smaller organizations of Western publishers such as the Council of Oriental Medical Publishers (COMP) have attempted to set standards and guidelines for translation in Chinese medicine, no administrative body has the power to enforce a standard in any translation at this time. Privilege and power are shifting roles and are not determined from "above." In the field of Chinese medicine, moreover, it is not a question of lack of access to knowledge, either Chinese language knowledge or translation knowledge. Access here is relatively even, despite the very uneven distribution of Chinese language knowledge that is often a conscious choice rather than an imposed disadvantage related to structural inequalities. Together with the lack of centralized authority, this makes for a very complex field when it comes to understanding the debates for and against standardization in Chinese medicine.

On one hand, there are those who take a cultural approach toward the debates over standardization. To help to reverse the culturally based biases that lead to distortions of original Chinese medical ideas, Wiseman thus argues that there needs to be clearly delineated source-oriented standards:

> To get people thinking about Chinese medicine in the way that Chinese physicians do, diagnosing in the way Chinese physicians do, and providing the treatment that Chinese physicians do, we need a set of terms where everything in the English is related to everything in the Chinese. In other words to transmit Chinese medical concepts faithfully, we need a standardized vocabulary pegged to Chinese (Wiseman 2000b: 20).

The call for a standardized terminology here is very much linked to the importance of faithfulness to the original concept. When these concepts are taken to be technical terms, moreover, faithfulness through standards becomes more critical. This argument thus classifies Chinese medical language as a "Language for Special Purposes" (LSP) that qualifies for a formal, standardized terminology (see also Kovacs 1989):

> Two fundamental criteria for distinguishing an LSP: a) its use is restricted to a social group involved with specific activities; b) its having a specific terminology relating the objects and concepts of the activity in question. It is notably on the basis of these two criteria that the language of Chinese medicine is unequivocally characterized as an LSP (Wiseman 2000c: 53).

Wiseman compares the language of Chinese medicine to the language of biomedicine and emphasizes that in the process of translating biomedicine into Chinese, the technical nature of the material was treated seriously. The material was thus translated according to the motive for transmission "to simply acquire the same understanding of the subject matter as the source community" (Wiseman 2001a: 19), a motivation that led to the supreme importance of source-oriented translation. Especially when the target audience consists of students, teachers, and practitioners, proponents of standardization argue, this issue becomes incredibly important. Many scholars and practitioners, in both the United States and China, concur with Wiseman in this regard, agreeing upon the need for source-oriented standards that honor the original, technical knowledge (Ergil 2001, 2006; Ergil and Ergil 2006; Felt 2000, 2006a, b; Flaws 2000, 2006a, b; Niu 2004; Rosenberg 2006). From this perspective, standardization is seen as a measure of protection for the Chinese. By instituting standards, translations will be able to convey more accurately the plurality in Chinese points of view rather than confusing them with Western moral frameworks and Western ideologies of language as arbitrary.

Proponents of standardization further draw upon the major issue of linguistic access to argue their case, especially in the context of students and clinicians of Chinese medicine:

> The use of a standard translational terminology pegged to the Chinese originals also makes it easier to learn to read the Chinese language literature in Chinese. In this case, one would only use a single dictionary or glossary to learn the meanings of the main words and compound terms (Flaws 2006a: 27).

This is an important issue, especially related to the view that language in Chinese medicine constitutes an access point of truth, where the only way into the heart of the original is through learning the original language, Chinese. "For those who 'broker' the practice of acupuncture in the United States," Emad notes, "the issue of cultural translation is deeply enmeshed in a debate over Chinese-language knowledge" (2006: 409). In this view, the only people who have access to the deep truths of Chinese medicine are those with access to the language, and only with a standardized translation can readers trust that they are being led back to the same source. Finally, the issue of academic freedom consistently resurfaces in the translation debates, where proponents of standardization argue that reader autonomy should constitute the freedom *not* to have to depend on any one translator's ideas in order to learn about Chinese medicine:

> Target-oriented translation that takes the form of bleaching out Chinese medical concepts by familiar expression or of deliberate omission tends to impose a personal interpretation. The reader gets only what the translator thinks is useful in Chinese medicine (Wiseman 2000c: 229).

In other words, Wiseman's view is that a standardized terminology forces translators to explain their term choices instead of leaving readers to depend on their whims.

There are many other reasons for standards that debate participants argue for. Firstly, it is argued that standardization is needed for accurate communication across texts and with other scholars and practitioners, especially as the field grows ever larger. Comparing standards in Chinese medicine with Mandarin Chinese, Ding (2006) points out that standards in Chinese makes communication possible. A related argument is that, for new authors, a standardized terminology would allow them immediately to tap into the language community, drawing upon established standards to create their text (Flaws 2006a: 17). Secondly, the issue of legitimacy is prominent in discussions about standardized Chinese medical language. Emphasizing the need for standard terminology to present Chinese medicine to outside parties "such as governmental and regulatory agencies, third party payers (insurance companies), CAM group practices, hospital administrators, and other potential employers," Flaws argues that we need to present a united front so that these organizations will see Chinese medicine as a system worth integrating (2006a: 17). Thirdly, the fact that "a standard professional terminology is also needed to research and access information digitally" has not gone unnoticed (Flaws 2006a: 17). For example, a patient or practitioner conducting an Internet search for a Chinese medical term under the current circumstances would be given an assortment of confusing and conflicting information. A standard, the argument goes, would facilitate the possibility of finding meaning amidst this confusion.

Several international organizations, such as the China-based World Federation of Chinese Medical Societies (WFCMS) and the Western Pacific Region of the World Health Organization (WHO-WPR), have hosted a series of international meetings to develop English language Chinese medical terminology standards. While the WFCMS is interested in developing these standards to enhance communication across the wide variety of traditional, biomedical, and integrative professional organizations that it interacts with, the WHO-WPR is invested in the standard terms so that they may be included in a section on traditional medicine of the upcoming eleventh edition of the International Classification of Diseases (ICD-11). This project has led to the 2007 release of the *WHO International Standard Terminologies on Traditional Medicine in the Western Pacific Region* (WHO-IST), a term list consisting of about four thousand traditional medical terms in Chinese and their English translations (WHO-WPR 2007). It is closely tied in with the overall WHO goal of creating an International Classification of Traditional Medicine (ICTM), complete with standard diagnostic codes, treatment strategies, and terminology based on "modern information sciences" (sites.google.com/site/whoictm/home). In the course of the five years that this study has been underway, this process has moved forth at incredible speeds, and the ICD-11 codes are imminent, although the extent to which they are actually based on the WHO-WPR standards is debatable.

The issues of communication, legitimacy, and digital access all coincide with the reasoning of the WHO and WFCMS in striving for standardization of English language Chinese medical terms. Official standards in the ICD-11, for example, would not only allow physicians of biomedicine and Chinese medicine to communicate more easily, but would also facilitate the communication between providers and insurance companies. Likewise, it would serve to put a professional face on the language of Chinese medicine in an international context and in so doing would boost the legitimacy of the field. Finally, the issue of digital access becomes crucial when dealing with an international and integrated digital health database, where not only patients, but providers and organizations as well, will need to have standard terms in order to connect. The WHO's goals for standardization differ significantly, however, from Wiseman and colleagues. As one anonymous poster wrote in a 2011 Listserve discussion about the recent ICTM efforts, the WHO standards are being created "for political reasons only," with no basis in academic principles of translation. For this reason, Wiseman and other scholars who otherwise strongly support standardization have removed themselves from the international efforts to standardize not only language in Chinese medicine, but also practice. Here, they align themselves with a perspective that insists on learning, as another poster comments, "what the words *mean*" rather than what a group of non-native English speakers, politicians moreover, agree on what the standard should be.

The notion of linguistic domination, by politicians, or for that matter, academicians, strikes a deep chord among practitioners and students in Chinese medicine, the majority of whom are opposed to any form of standardization. The idea of authors being forced to use a standard language not of their own choice seems to go against the freedom characterizing American culture. From this perspective, standardization of terms is a form of dominance and *both* Wiseman and the WHO are attempting to become hegemonic leaders. "While appropriate for a church aspiring to doctrinal hegemony over the faithful, such a dogma is not suited to a community engaged in propagating a complex, eclectic medical system, itself in a continuous process of evolution and adaptation" (Beinfield and Korngold 2001: 146). Following this view, standardization of terms is also a form of censorship. With a standard in place, participants argue, "communications would have had to squeeze through a terminological hiatus created and policed by an elite few who understood the root terminology" (Buck 2000: 39). In this sense, opponents of standardization in Chinese medicine subscribe to the notion of standardized, "proper" language as associated with power, authority, and dominance (Bourdieu 1991; Gal 1989; Woolard 1998). Standardized language, from this perspective, is a measure of control, of power based on the "structural disparity between the very unequal *knowledge* of the legitimate language and the much more uniform *recognition* of this language" (Bourdieu 1991: 62). To many in the field of Chinese medicine, then, standardization from any direction is equivalent to social control.

In a related argument, opponents of standardization also insist that plurality in translation reflects the plurality of Chinese medical theories in China, where "Chinese medical literature was written, in the course of 2000 years, by innumerable authors with different ideas and world views" (Beinfield and Korngold 2001: 149). "This richness," they continue, "appears to be reproducible in translations only if those who produce those renderings also start from different perspectives themselves" (Beinfield and Korngold 2001: 149). Beinfield and Korngold thus invoke the long history of different interpretations in Chinese medicine to make the claim that such plurality should also naturally characterize English translations. Beyond the multiplicity of theories, the terms themselves are also understood to convey an inherent plurality that standard terminology erases. If the meanings of Chinese medical terms have shifted so many times over two thousand years, there is no way to capture the many Chinese meanings in one English term (Bensky et al. 2006; Shen 2006; Shima 2006). In addition to arguing that more than one English term for a single Chinese medical word "does not necessarily obscure its meaning," these scholars therefore suggest that "the rigid application of the principle of one to one correspondence in translating Chinese terms into English easily oversimplifies Chinese medical ideas" (Bensky et al. 2006: 14). Standard English terms, in this case, are seen as limiting the possibilities of meaning that Chinese words carry.

Opponents of standardization also argue that source-oriented translation leads to terms that are difficult to understand and use. Asking "[D]o we want a highly technical language that separates us from our patients in the way Latin does in modern medicine?" (Deadman 2000: 56), they thus advocate for a simpler language that captures the essential beauty and nonlinearity of Chinese words, a beauty that is lost in a scientized technical language (Chinese medical instructor, 2005, personal communication). This view is further reinforced by the notion that Chinese words used in Chinese medicine are actually not specialized, but are common. "Ordinary words in Chinese are often adopted as technical terms in the context of Chinese medicine to convey specialist meanings" (Buck 2000: 38). The ordinariness of Chinese medical terms in the context of their culture seems a logical case for the argument that the corresponding English language terms should also be ordinary and familiar.

As briefly mentioned above, a further issue related to this particular view is the ambivalence about language and the idea that language is not as important as clinical or personal experience in learning or thinking about Chinese medical ideas. In this view, scholars of language are by their very nature different from practitioners and cannot know the truths of practice. "Difficulties arise," Buck explains, "because the professional imperatives incumbent upon linguistic scholars differ somewhat from the requirements of Chinese medical practitioners and educators" (2000: 40). Indeed, as Ho (2006) found, the notion that Chinese medical concepts are not intelligible in language is common in the United States, especially with concepts such as *qi*. Ho goes on to explain how, despite the experiential component, practitioners had no problem talking about *qi* in English (Ho 2006: 422). According to opponents of standardization, such ability to talk about and explain *qi* would be severely limited by the requirements of an imposed standardized language. Fratkin thus posits that "the attempt by some publishers to 'insist' that everyone, including the Chinese, use Wiseman translations is wrong, and it emanates from intellectual snobbery" and that "it unfortunately pits Chinese language academics against clinicians" (2006: 22). Thus, as Wiseman laments, the separation between "scholarship" and "practice" has become a commonplace trope in American Chinese medical circles.

An overarching concern affecting all sides of the standardization debate is the issue of clinical and educational relevance. For example, one of the major reasons that many scholars argue for a source-oriented and standardized approach to translation is that it makes a difference for students and clinicians who will use the material to treat suffering individuals. Citing cases where multiple Chinese words for a type of symptom or illness pattern, such as pain or diarrhea, are translated into a single English term that does not differentiate between the multiple concepts originally represented in Chinese, such scholars argue that lack of term standards leads to a decline in clinical efficacy (Ergil 2001; Ergil and Ergil 2006; Felt 2006a; Wiseman 2000c, 2002a). They also point out that when different authors use different terms, cross-referencing books and relating them back to the original Chinese becomes impossible:

> When multiple terms are used and the reader has no way to determine what the original term was, he then has no way of understanding that each of the terms represents the same idea. Not only does the meaning of the original character get lost in the shuffle, but new ideas emerge and become a part of the corpus of information that makes up traditional Chinese medicine for the English speaker. Anthropologically this is an extremely interesting phenomenon. From the point of view of a clinician however, it can change the nature of a clinically significant idea and create a great deal of confusion (Ergil 2001: 7).

As Ergil here observes, the changes taking place within Chinese medicine as they are translated to a U.S. context are anthropologically interesting, but they can also impact the effective transmission of clinical Chinese medicine as it is practiced in China. The practitioners in the United States thereby become less effective than are their Chinese counterparts. Other scholars suggest that rather than strive for standardization or precision in the translation of educational texts, using a multiplicity of terms in this context creates a "terminological chaos" that actually benefits students as they learn to negotiate the depths of Chinese medical concepts (Bensky et al. 2006; Chase 2006; Mitchell 2006). They further suggest that the labeling of terms is irrelevant to the student's ability to "know what it feels like and what it means" (Maciocia 2000: 51).

Students' perspectives on standardization are also complex, textured by the shifting territory inherent in trying to integrate a new language into personal systems of meaning. In this sense, ideas and feelings about standardization are mapped—through multiple specific moments of engagement—onto each person's basic experience of meaning in Chinese medicine. Like the general population in the United States, students resist the notion that such a personal process could ever be mediated by a remote group of "experts." At times of frustration and confusion, however, they crave a coherent, quick gloss for terms that seem to have an endless array of definitions and explanations, none of which are clear in English. As they proceed through the program, they begin to get a sense of how much easier communication between practitioners would become if they all spoke a common language, but they also recognize that something might be lost if such a language were to come at the cost of the multiplicity in translations that gives them a shadowy yet somehow more vivid picture of the richness of meaning in Chinese. In their final years of study, students often come away with a certain ambivalence toward standardization, a recognition of the ways in which it would help as well as the ways in which it would hurt. But American students, with their particular concerns and priorities, the issue is never quite as personal as the process of learning how to *use* language in the effort to become an effective and compassionate healer.

From this detailed discussion, it is clear that ideologies of standardization in the translation of Chinese medicine are both diverse and complex. The arguments overlap with conversations about standardization in linguistic anthropology and translation studies more generally, and yet the differences are significant. Firstly, generally speaking, there is not necessarily a so-called privileged class to speak of in the Chinese medicine language debates. Most, if not all, of the participants in the debates are highly educated, middle-class scholars and clinicians. This leads to complications when we try to apply anthropological theories of power, hegemony, and the marginalized classes. Secondly, and related to the first point, is the lack of any centralized authority dominating the standard language that should be used for translation in Chinese medicine. The WHO certainly suggests such an authority, but the interpretation of what exactly this means in the context of Chinese medical translation is anything but clear. Although resistance to dominance by a centralized authority is just as rampant in Chinese medicine as it is elsewhere in the world, at the present time such an authority is far from dominant. Moreover, because it is challenging popular notions of translation in Chinese medicine (evidenced by most teachers and educators), the authority can in this case actually be considered a type of resistance. Thirdly, plurality within the context of the debates refers to the freedom to translate Chinese words in different ways depending on the experience and creativity of the author (Beinfield and Korngold 2001). As such, it does represent the type of multiplicity in ways of speaking that linguistic ideology studies strive to capture. In this case, however, multiplicity is grounded in ideologies based on what some anthropologists would call an essentialized notion of culture and language, which is a view that linguistic anthropologists often strive to offset by introducing the need for recognition of diversity. Ideologies for or against standardization in the translation of Chinese medicine are therefore complex, and this complexity often mediates the enactment of translation in everyday practice.

Section Discussion

In this section, I have discussed various ideologies of translation in Chinese medicine, drawing mostly upon professional and scholarly participants' perspectives to demonstrate the diversity of views on translation. As with ideologies of language, ideologies of translation are also intimately related to the multiple historical, institutional, moral, and material realities surrounding Chinese medicine in China and the United States. Again, they are also deeply tied to traditional Western ways of understanding language as referential, language as culture, and language as a tool.

Conclusion

In this chapter, I have discussed many different ideologies of language and ideologies of translation in Chinese medicine: language as arbitrary, language as determinative of thought, language as a tool, language as cultural capital, translation as transfer, translation as a tool of power, translation as im/possible, and translation standards as un/necessary. As we move on to look at the ways in which translation in Chinese medicine is actually enacted—through inscription, interaction, embodied experience, and practice—it is important to keep these ideologies in mind. I will reiterate here the importance of viewing such ideologies not as inflexible or mutually exclusive ways of thinking, but as adaptable perspectives that are available to all who participate in the translation of Chinese medicine in any form. As such, these ideologies function as mediators rather than determiners of the enactment of translation. Alongside history, institutional frameworks, moral frameworks, and material objects, they work—indeed, they often *play*—together as participants move in and out of their experiences writing, reading, learning, and practicing Chinese medicine in translation.

CHAPTER 3

Living Inscription in Chinese Medicine

For an idea to be included in the canon of Chinese medical theory, it needs to be around for hundreds of years. It's not going to be officially a part of the canon of Chinese medicine until it's withstood the test of time, kay? This is in contrast to if you're writing a paper for a modern Western audience, you need to quote the latest data. If you're writing a paper and you're trying to make your point—in Chinese—let's say you're writing a book and you want to introduce a concept? You will quote the classics. You will quote the Neijing.

—Carter, instructor in first-year Fundamentals of Oriental Medicine course

This chapter begins the in-depth examination of the enactment of translation in Chinese medicine by looking specifically at inscriptions—texts—as they are mediated by the diverse historical, institutional, and moral circumstances of both author and audience. Although the focus is on the enactment of translation through writing, the notion of living translation lies at the heart of this discussion. And so while Ricœur argues that texts must be approached as fixed records wherein meaning is detached from the original, fleeting situation and cemented in a written form (Ricœur 1976), in this chapter I discuss how texts in Chinese medicine can also productively be approached rather as an "architecture of social relations" (Silverstein and Urban 1996: 14). Far from being a rigid sedimentation of abstract ideas, textuality in Chinese medicine is "a mode of social action" (Hanks 1989: 103) in which author-practitioners simultaneously draw upon their experience as well as the work of past scholar-physicians to respond to other texts, communicate with future practitioners, and create innovative practices. In this sense, textuality is approached by participants as a personally meaningful "social relation" (Farquhar 1994: 206) that is intensely mediated by historical and institutional, moral, and ideological landscapes. Through both interdiscursitvity, understood as the mixing of genres, discourses, or styles (Fairclough 1992; Wu 2011), and intertexuality, understood as the interpellation of texts with pieces of other texts (Fairclough 1992; Kristeva 1980), textual products of living translation thus unfold as a set of "conversations" that authors carry on with real and imagined original authors, as well as readers, students, and patients. These conversations further work to encode the language of Chinese medicine in multiple formats that themselves carry on the process of living translation through their publication and consumption, variably reproducing the practice of Chinese medicine through the mediated mixing of genres and styles of talk and the intermixing of strategically selected historical texts.

The process of mapping these conversations becomes important here, primarily because the living nature of textuality in Chinese medicine only begins with the way the texts are written. It continues in the social life of the texts and the way they are taken up, the way texts themselves are engaged with as objects of consumption (Boyarin 1993; Eco 1979; Iser 1978; Poulet 1969; Ricoeur 1976; Sterponi 2004, 2007). This perspective complicates the traditional boundaries separating text from nontext, as "extratextual" factors permeate the interpretation and use of texts along sometimes unexpected lines (Hanks 1989). For scholars of translation who focus mostly on texts, it opens up the possibility of looking at the entire enterprise of publication in Chinese medicine as a continuous, creative event where people are involved in a set of conversations that are themselves indexes of living history. What is especially relevant in Chinese medicine is that the translated material is also enacted upon living bodies as healing practice.

From this vantage point, the "living" nature of textuality and translation in Chinese medicine involves multiple participants in an ongoing stream of interaction wherein the living, breathing practice of medicine is always and constantly engaged with the written record. In crafting new translations, each author is indeed interdiscursively engaging in a "scribal culture" (Montgomery 2000) that extends from China to the United States to Europe and beyond, and spans thousands of years of discourse and practice. Participation in this community, especially as a translator creating texts for particular American English-speaking audiences, demands an engagement with key controversial questions and ideologies of language and translation, discussed extensively in the last two chapters. The issue of faithfulness or fidelity, for example, requires translators to choose, on some level, between either a source-oriented or a target-oriented approach. Likewise, the question of terminology standardization requires translators either to commit to translating consistently or include a multitude of terminologies in a single text. The question of biomedicalization forces translators to negotiate the boundaries of medical systems, to police them with terminology, or to blur them in language that clearly seeks to integrate worldviews. And the thorny question of commensurability and linguistic relativity challenges translators to take a stand on what they even consider to be possible in translation.

As described above, these are not just linguistic issues. The infinite partiality of textual interdiscursivity reverberates in every choice that authors make when it comes to what aspects of the networks of textual traditions they nurture in translation. When it comes to creating texts, then, translation is a deeply moral issue linked to the respect one proffers on to the source culture or author vis-à-vis the language one uses to faithfully (or unfaithfully) reproduce the work in another context. As Judith Farquhar (1994) notes, in Chinese medicine, it is also a personal and social issue, as past authors and physicians are approached as teachers with whom one develops an intimate relationship. The questions of terminology standardization, biomedicalization, and commensurability are also equally embedded in the everyday social, cultural, personal, and moral life-worlds of participants, made all the more complicated by the fact that, in the living textuality of Chinese medicine, there are always multiple sources, multiple targets, and multiple ongoing conversations.

In this chapter, we enter directly into the stream of these conversations, observing how different authors and translators approach the "mangle of practice" (Pickering 1995; see also Scheid 2002) that is textuality in Chinese medicine. The nature of this living textuality is described in the first section, whereas the second section describes some of the challenges faced by professional translators when they attempt to transmit Chinese medical knowledge in text form, including especially how the inherent *interdiscursivity* of texts in Chinese medicine challenges them to create so-called authentic translations. The second section of the chapter looks at a single term, 魄 *po,* that is translated as "corporeal soul," "animal soul," or "vigor," depending on the author. Through a detailed examination of seven explanations of *po,* paired with public statements on translation ideologies, I demonstrate the many ways in which each translation of even a single term emerges as an inscription of the complex, morally and socially grounded interrelationship(s) among author, original, and audience. This perspective shows how the moral frameworks as well as the epistemologies of language and translation explored in the last two chapters come to life in the real-world practice of creating texts for reader consumption in specific historical and institutional settings. It further shows how a single Chinese term is translated over time in multiple texts. I conclude with a discussion of how this view on living inscription in the enactment of translation in Chinese medicine invites us into an examination of the complex links between textual translation and everyday interpretation, including practice.

Living Textuality in Chinese Medicine

Chinese medicine, wherever it is practiced, is a deeply textual tradition. This section describes the nature of this textuality, including a discussion of the vast range of texts in Chinese medicine, both in China as well as in translation.

In contrast to biomedicine, where even the most recent textbooks are considered suspect because of the rapidly changing knowledge in the field (Konner 1987: 14–15), classical texts are held in high esteem in Chinese medicine. Such "classics," memorized and recopied over hundreds of years, are considered canonical and authoritative, as Carter, the first-year teacher quoted at the outset of this chapter, observes. Furth describes these classics as "works of high antiquity believed to express universal truths about the universe, human society, and ethics—truths that flowed inevitably from their status as canon" (2007b: 125). These classic treatises, including the *Huangdi Nei Jing* (Yellow Emperor's Classic), the *Nan Jing* (The Classic of Difficult Issues), the *Shanghan Lun* (Treatise on Cold Damage), the *Shennong Bencao* (Shennong's Herbal Classic), among many others, are often understood to be compilations themselves constructed by many authors over time:

> Many ancient medical classics are unreadable until they have been collated. They were copied and recopied by many hands, handed down generation to generation, and spread to many places. Mistakes were unavoidable (Ma 1989: 10).

Additionally, there are multiple versions of commentary texts in which scholar-practitioners from different times and places interpret the often quite sparse and ambiguous classical material. Rather than straightforward translations, however, commentaries are also opportunities for later authors to generate innovative strategies for utilizing classical wisdom in treating patients. "The openness of commentary," argues Furth, "lies in the way it both calls attention to a privileged authority and signals its own distance from that authority" (2007b: 132). As Karchmer explains, "To become a virtuouso Chinese medicine doctor is to learn how to 'make a text your own'" (2004: 219). Commentators as well as individual practitioners who draw upon multiple texts thus make the classics their own through reflection, practice, and further extended commentary. The classic texts in Chinese medicine are thus simultaneously authoritative and open to interpretation, at once grounded in an inscribed "chain of authentication" (Agha 2007: 218) and yet innovative at the same time. The practice of "intralingual" or within-language translation (Jakobson 1966 [1959]) is thus a key part of textuality in Chinese medicine, where multiple authors make the texts their own through a translation within the source language itself. In this sense, Chinese classical texts can be understood themselves as "landscapes" of possibility (Yamada 1999; as cited by Suh 2013).

In addition to classical texts, the case study genre of text is "as old as medicine itself," or so says a recent mainland Chinese textbook (Furth 2007b: 126). In case study texts, individual physicians provide evidence in the form of specific illness events, usually describing the symptoms, the diagnosis and prognosis, the treatment, and the (often positive) results. As a venue for creative thinking, Furth explains that the case study genre offers physicians a unique outlet:

> In the dialectic between text and experience, producing medical knowledge using cases privileged the latter, allowing physicians to bypass the traditional canon/commentary mode of thinking common in classics and historical learning for a direct consideration of clinical manifestations (Furth 2007a: 14).

Even still, in case studies it is common practice to cite specific passages from canonical texts in the performance of expert knowledge, again intralingually translating past knowledge through the lens of clinical experience.

As more formal training programs arose during the Communist era, textbooks as opposed to classical texts with commentaries began to play "an even more significant role in the development of Chinese medicine, not just stabilizing a new paradigm but also actively participating in its creation" (Karchmer 2004: 143–144). Even in textbook form, however, the classic texts are quoted liberally and foundationally, often overtly cultivating "the sense of a glorious, unbroken intellectual tradition and clinical expertise dating to the legendary Yellow Emperor" as a way of "establishing credibility" (Lo 2009: 290). In similar fashion, the many newsletters, pamphlets, and popular texts on Chinese medicine today are each constructed as a simultaneous conversation with the documented past of Chinese medicine, as well as with the desired future. Chinese medical texts are further in constant conversation with the daily practice of acupuncture, prescription, massage, and, in the last one hundred years, biomedicine. In the case of many of the classics, they are written as dialogues between an expert and novice, overtly geared toward the generation of practice. More modern texts are conspicuously created by physicians and acupuncturists in dialogue with colleagues in both Chinese and biomedicine. In many cases, they are also crafted intentionally as handbooks to be picked up, quoted, and used to explain treatment approaches and clinical action. Books and other documents are also often created as sociopolitical devices to demonstrate the legitimacy of Chinese medicine vis-à-vis scientific biomedicine. Here, for example, biomedicine's reliance on experimentation and anatomical knowledge has challenged Chinese medicine to validate its claims on truth, illness, and the body.

In many ways, then, the epistemological diversity of textuality in Chinese medicine is similar to the situation of modern Ayurveda, where "in addition to the strand of rational empiricism, there is also an equal valuing of foundational truths codified in text as well as of the practitioner's own subjective experience" (Wolfgram 2010: 151). Within this "epistemologically hybrid" environment, contemporary participants often use language strategically to draw upon these multiple epistemologies to position Ayurveda in the contemporary world (Wolfgram 2010: 152). Authors in Chinese medicine arguably participate in the same epistemological game when they variably highlight different aspects of textual and personal knowledge as valid.

In this sense, texts in Chinese medicine are richly interdiscursive. They are invariably built "with respect to other text occasions" (Silverstein 1996: 81). Each text in Chinese medicine, even each term, is not only oriented toward a host of other texts (see Bauman 2004), but is also "multiply dialogical" (Irvine 1996: 151) as specific authors explain the meaning of illness concepts by weaving a network of quotes from classic and modern texts into a particular inscription. In so doing, they simultaneously use interdiscursivity as a legitimation strategy (Crapanzano 2011) as well as contributing to and participating in an elaborate conversation that spans both space and time. Within this network, specialized Chinese medical terminology, built out of complex Chinese characters and combinations of characters, accumulates its characteristic polysemy and heteroglossia.

So far I have been discussing only Chinese texts. English translations of Chinese medicine, as in Chinese, include direct translations of classics, translations of commentaries and case study texts, and original English-language commentaries on translations of commentaries. There are compilations of secondary translations, spiral-bound teacher-organized texts, and original texts introducing Chinese medicine to students, patients, and the public. As in Chinese, there are also scholarly journals, newsletters, and pamphlets. Each of these translations regularly organizes itself around a series of quotes from classic Chinese texts, sometimes gathering such material from other translations and sometimes from original sources. Many of the English texts are also written as guides to clinical practice and most discuss Chinese medical concepts in terms of their biomedical "Others." Body parts and functions are thus commonly held up to widely accepted biomedical notions of anatomy and physiology, and the differences between them become the foundation for a kind of philosophical, moral positioning that elaborates on biomedicine's perceived reductionism and Chinese medicine's inherent holism (see chapter 1). In other texts, Chinese medicine is lauded as a scientific practice that complements but does not challenge biomedicine. As in Chinese, then, each English-language text in Chinese medicine is a richly intertextual inscription of multiple, continuous conversations with past, present, and future actors, each with complex allegiances to various political, moral, and cultural communities of practice.

Each translated text is also, I might add, an entextualization of a multiply dialogic and heteroglossic, deeply moral, personal, and social conversation that unfolds between the author-translator and the original, no matter what kind of original or set of originals is imagined. In this sense, the writing of Chinese medical texts, whether they are direct translations or adaptations, is first constituted by the ways in which particular authors approach and understand the Chinese material, especially the way they tackle its inherent intertextuality and interdiscursivity, its embeddedness in thousands of years of Chinese texts and practice, and its complex relationship with biomedicine. Translated texts are also necessarily created in dialogue with other English-language texts, with the other authors they seek to complement or contrast, and of course, always with the scientific biomedical paradigm they either seek to challenge, contrast, or to support. Finally, each text is also created as a conversation between the author-translator and his or her imagined audience, with their desires, their demands, and their language always shaping translation decisions. In all of these cases, the crafting of texts is undertaken with particular strategies, particular ideologies of what it means to translate authentically, what it means to heal, what it means to be historically or clinically accurate, and what it means to be hopeful about the future of medicine and healthcare. Inscriptions emerge from the answers to such questions, and original material is reinscribed with particular values as well as particular affective, epistemic, and moral stances in the process. Furthermore, not every text is equally interdiscursive with every community, and authors must choose who to talk to and what about, which of the multiple sources and multiple targets they want to engage, and the type of practice they seek to generate. Translators also have to work consciously to establish their own authority within these communities, their very right to translate, through various kinds of evidence. The texts themselves can thus be approached as indices of the living practice that is Chinese medicine. As such, living translation is already, even at the "static" level of text, a conversation in motion.

Involved Inscriptions

When a translator of Chinese medicine, driven by the desire to create a new system of healing or to transmit accurately a foreign knowledge-base, sets out on the long road that eventually leads to a book, she faces a series of complex challenges. This section describes some of these challenges and discusses the ways in which various translators have enacted solutions through their work. Based on ethnographic interviews with translators in the United States, Europe, Taiwan, and China, the section includes comments from translators struggling with interdiscursivity and intertextuality, book formatting, language and morality, and the balance between the need to find resonance with original material at the same time as with anticipated audiences.

First and foremost, there is the problem of trying to transmit knowledge that is already entrenched in a complex web of interdiscursivity spanning hundreds of years of practice and scholarship. Especially when working with the translation of classical Chinese texts, authors are not only faced with finding

English equivalents for the grammatically complex, extremely sparse, and often ambiguous classical Chinese language, but they also face the challenge presented by the fact that classical Chinese differs significantly depending upon the era in which it was written. A European translator explains:

> You know, if I concentrate on *Shanghan Lun,* and then the *Nanjing, Lingshu,* this very old stuff, and then I did stuff from Zhang Jingyue. I did stuff from *Shuijing Lun,* and more in the nineteenth century, and doing modern stuff as well. And that is my major problem is that I'm—I'm not specialized in any period. So now I'm doing the *Shanghan* from Cheng Wuji, and I think, wow, Jesus, you know, these are—you know, not, not, not really the terminology. I can find my way now in terminology; I can solve things. But the, the surrounding language, the literary language, classical language, can be very different from author to author. That's one of the major things that, um, that's still troubling me. You know? And I always tell myself, yeah, you should have read more, but yeah, I did other things in life.

In working on texts from different time periods and different authors, this translator faces the difficulty of navigating period-specific language that tests the boundaries of his specialization and shames him into the feeling that to translate accurately, he should first have read the whole complex web of texts that might be referred to in any given single text he is trying to translate.

This complexity motivates many translators toward a full-speed plunge into the interdiscursive web of classic texts and contemporary commentaries. They endeavor to read everything, to know intimately each commentator and to study each character closely to capture it fully in all its dialogic significance and to find an equivalent that matches and explains all of it most precisely. As one translator puts it, it becomes a matter of "fidelity" and "faithfulness" to create texts that authentically reflect what Chinese people are and were doing at the time the original was created:

> I wanted to study Chinese medicine as it was practiced by Chinese people, and as it was experienced by Chinese people in Chinese society.

For many of the translators I interviewed, to access this kind of authentic practice, to bridge this cultural divide, a deeply involved scholarly practice is thus necessary.

This can be a frustrating process, however, as not even modern Chinese texts offer this type of comprehensive review of any given classical treatise. Another European translator explains:

> Like I read the Chinese—I read the *Qianjin Fang,* the Chinese editions of it. And the footnotes are crap, because the people that write them haven't read the other ten texts that pertain to that particular text at that time.

Without even a solid Chinese foundation to rest their translations upon, then, American and European translators creating texts in English have to proceed in what another translator likens to an "academic vacuum" in which self-driven decisions abound. In this sense, the inherent intertextuality and rich interdiscursivity of Chinese medical texts demands translators to become involved, to learn themselves how to listen to their source authors with an intensity that might be lessened by a more fixed target. Through an in-depth "sensori-motor, interpretive and emotional involvement" with textuality (Sterponi 2004: 1), translators thus embark on their translation quests as an ongoing search for a sense of resonance that often, given the complexity of the material, seems quite slippery. As a result, they often work together in workshops and less formal meetings to plunge the depths of Chinese language and history, forging translations that aim to achieve this particular form of cultural accuracy.

Such complexity in Chinese medical translation can be particularly challenging even for translators working to translate contemporary or modern clinical texts, in which many classical quotes are often embedded. These quotes, which can number as many as ten in a single paragraph, are mostly in various forms of classical Chinese, usually about one to three lines. The realization of this challenge is often something that only emerges over time for many translators, however, who begin with a simplified notion that being able to read modern Chinese will suffice for translating Chinese medicine, at least contemporary texts and articles. They soon discover, however, that they need a whole lot more background preparation, more reading of classical texts, and more study of writing styles to explain even one quote in one modern text. For obvious reasons, time limitations and clinical priorities being major factors, not everyone does all of this background study.

The way each translator handles the slipperiness of interdiscursivity and intertextuality in Chinese medicine is intimately intertwined with who she is, what she is trying to create with her translation, and who she is trying to reach. The whole project, as an entextualization of her own search for resonance, is a quest for a connection to the Other as well as it is a seeking out of a reasonable evidential basis strong enough to support her translation choices. This search emerges not only in conversation with all of the Chinese texts, and all the complexity indexed therein, but also in conversation with the entire existing library of English-language texts. For many translators, then, an initial engagement with existing translations, a realization that they are in some way lacking, sparks their desire to translate. Upon starting his own training in Chinese medicine in Europe, for example, one translator notes that "it was immediately apparent to me that, ah, the information [in the available translated texts] was flawed." For another translator, the information was not necessarily flawed so much as it was unsatisfactory in the sense of not being clear about what was a translation and what was an explanation based on the author's experience. For many budding scholars, this raises the question of accuracy. In the words of yet another translator:

> At a cursory glance I realized, uh-oh, if we really translate Chinese medicine in, ah, *faithfully*, then we're going to end up with something quite different from what was contained in those English books that we were looking at.

This scholar goes on to note that the biomedicalized, simplified translation of Chinese medicine contained in the English books he began looking at was, simply, inaccurate. For him, this is a moral issue leading him to judge available translations in terms of their authentic historical meaning. This realization conveys a sort of burden upon the author, a moral responsibility to translate more faithfully, without simplification. For this particular translator, there was some element of emotionality involved in this assessment:

> I was—is there a mild version of the word contemptuous? You know? Why do they do it like that? Why are they, you know, so cavalier with Chinese concepts? Why do they simplify everything?

Clearly, there is an affective component to this author's stance, a mild scorn or disdain for the transgression committed by other translators at the time. His life work has thus become to contribute to an ever-growing library of traditional translations.

For others, however, looking at available English translations leads to the sense that they are by far too traditional, not clearly scientific enough to put Chinese medicine in the running for mainstream medical status. Many Chinese translators whom I interviewed, for example, argue instead for an increased interdiscursivity with respect to scientific biomedical discourses. From this perspective, true resonance is to be found in scientific epistemology, based in an abstract equivalence of body parts and symptoms, as well as daily practice in real-life integrative clinics. Many of the Chinese translators I interviewed felt especially strongly about this, and often argued this point. For them, translations need to reflect accurately the way Chinese medicine is used in current hospital practice. As one translator puts it, translations that use arcane language to talk about Chinese medicine make it inaccessible and unnecessarily complex:

> You still need a re-translation, to fill in the explanation. A translation, the best translation, you should look at it and immediately know what he is trying to say. Because translation is taking a message from one language and transmitting to another language. You want [your readers] to be able to look at this thing of yours and know—I say cup, this is cup. They know this is cup. If you use something else to say it, people won't understand. The first time seeing it, they should understand. That's the best translation.

He does admit that there are some terms in Chinese medicine that require a complex understanding of classical theory to translate. "But," he says, "this is another matter entirely." What should happen, especially for the basic terms that have a foundation in a universal human trait (like "ass," as one translator defiantly offers as an example), is that translations should be immediately recognizable and should reflect genuine integrative practice:

> Look at society developing. If you go to a TCM hospital for treatment of an illness, all you will hear are Western medical words. Bronchitis, they say "bronchitis" right? If they say you have pneumonia, they say "pneumonia."

"They" (the *real* people practicing medicine) use "bronchitis" to describe bronchitis and "pneumonia" to describe pneumonia. In other words, they think and speak, as this translator himself does, of biomedical disease categories and prescribe Chinese herbs and other medicinal substances according to a pattern within that disease. Genuine institutional practice and a common physiological basis are therefore the measures that this translator uses to judge an authentic and good translation. Like many of the other Chinese translators with whom I spoke, this translator also underscores the importance of scientific basis for translation. For these translators as well as the several Americans who also emphasize a scientific approach to translation, there is an element of wanting to make sure that critically positioned experts, namely Western biomedical physicians and scientists in positions of power, easily understand what the author is talking about. This way, Chinese medicine can be authentically translated into a global, mainstream medical discourse. The search for resonance, here, is thus also a search for recognition.

The prominence of biomedical discourses of the body, illness, and health in translations of Chinese medicine brings our attention to another social "layer" that drives much of text production in Chinese medicine. This layer involves the relationships and the dialogues that each author conducts with both imagined and real audiences. In the field of Chinese medicine, readers are not some faraway, unknown group, although there might always be some anonymous consumers of the texts. Far more present in the writing of texts are the students and colleagues who not only read the texts, but discuss them on Internet Listserves, who come to the two or three major professional conferences each year to hear authors speak and who find the authors to talk with in the hallways and among the many booths selling acupuncture needles, books, and herbal products at these conferences. So even while many translators agree that a more precise, standard terminology might help propel Chinese medicine into the category of "real medicine" as perceived by organizations like the WHO, they also know their readers. They know the way they already speak and the terminology they are comfortable with. They also know that they are heartily opposed, on principle, to anyone else dictating their language. The project of "finding themselves" (Van Hoy 2010) demands a certain creativity that they insist on getting from the books they read, and authors, many of whom are in full agreement, deliver.

For a large number of American translators, then, true resonance can only be found in their own clinical and personal experience. This experience becomes the evidence needed for certain translations. For one author, it is linked to the complex social project of addressing a particular set of disturbances and demands for self-improvement in American society. In this case, there is a distinct lack of regard for generating even the pretense that the material is a faithful representation of any original. Instead, in the attempt to "create a medicine" this translator attempts to be "honest" in his portrayal of the material as his own thoughts:

> So what I tried to do is create a medicine. I wasn't really trying to have powerful fidelity to anything. I wasn't representing myself as representing the thoughts of any of the people who I translated. Um, I was honest. And I feel many of the other translators aren't honest.

For this writer, who despite his lack of fidelity still considers himself a kind of translator of Chinese medicine, "faithfulness" is not especially high on his list of priorities. Instead, he is driven by the goal of creating a medicine that vibes with what he is doing on a daily basis in the clinic:

> I took full responsibility for what I was writing, and I openly admitted that this is my agenda. I'm ignoring everything in Chinese history that doesn't confirm it, and I'm selecting that which does to make a case for what I'm actually doing on a day-to-day basis in the treatment room. So everything I wrote reflects how I think about what I'm doing, or at least how I did at the time I wrote the books. But it was all authentic. It was all a living expression of what I was actually doing. And I think it's very dishonest to translate ancient texts under the pretense that you're conveying the values of the person who wrote them.

Responsibility in translation is clearly important for this scholar. Instead of the responsibility being to reproduce a certain kind of original meaning, text, or conversation, however, responsibility here is conceived as an honest expression of "living" practice. A translation is authentic, from this standpoint, if it directly reflects the values with which the author practices on a daily basis. On this basis, the translation of texts "under the pretense that you're conveying the values of the person who wrote them" is dishonest, as it neglects to mention the inevitable role of the translator's values in shaping the text. This translator thinks such values are central to the task of translation, which in his case is no less grand than the creation of a new medicine. In contrast to other English-language texts and authors who advocate for an increased scholarly appreciation of the dialogic nature of individual terms, and also in contrast to the argument that translation should be conducted in direct conversation with biomedical science, he argues firmly for an increased interdiscursivity with respect to what some might call a more New Age daily practice and desired future.

This commitment to New Age medical futures is for this author deeply linked to the notion of "integrity," and a certain idea of language:

> A true, *deep* quality of care that comes from the soul for the soul of another. Language can only be in service of that—language is not primary. So I say it's the most highly developed capacity, why? Because it allows us to *transmit* an authentic human experience to another human being who may be listening authentically. But if the authenticity isn't there, none of it matters. I would argue that people like Nigel Wiseman are just bright guys with a lot of big ideas and not much depth. And you can put that in print.

For this author, then, depth in service of humanity, care coming from the soul of one to another, is the purpose of language and of translation. This is clearly a strongly felt, deeply moral ideology of language as personal integrity that positions this author in direct and conscious opposition to several of the main debate participants who argue for standard translations. It is also a language ideology consistent with the views of many of his readers, as shown in the previous chapter, and he is acutely aware of this fact.

So far, I have shown several diverse, morally situated ways of approaching translation, each of them embedded deeply in an interdiscursive engagement with the imagined past of Chinese medicine, the present experience of the authors, and the anticipated experience of future readers. I have shown that each is mediated by the historical, institutional, and moral frameworks as well as the ideologies of language and translation that are available in the field. So while one translator may argue for more engagement with the classical past, another advocates increased dialogue with mainstream biomedical contexts. Yet another claims that to be genuinely authentic, translations must emerge from a more developed understanding of self. These views present a range of solutions for finding a resonant language to present Chinese medicine in English, and they are certainly some of the most common. But there are still other ways to approach the translation of Chinese medicine in texts. One author with whom I spoke, for example, refuses to engage with the translation debates entirely, arguing that authentic translations must convey the way each concept fits into the "system" of Chinese medicine. He thus claims that the basis for translation, rather than being the way a text reflects upon classics, biomedicine, or anything else, should be the understanding of how each concept fits into the "entire picture" of Chinese medicine:

> And, um, I mean for me this whole—the whole translation thing is—it's too kind of *word*—individual word focused … I have to try to figure a way to say this, but (pause) when you come to a character or a *term*—Let's just say an English term. Um, where there's debatable ways to translate it. You know, *ming men*—it could be life gate or gate of vitality, whatever. The real problem is not necessarily, in my opinion, um, a lack of understanding of exactly what the Chinese term is in the English term? … It's more of a lack of understanding of how the concept fits into the entire picture of, you know, the system of Chinese medicine.

In this excerpt, this translator examines the various ways in which a specific concept, 命门 *ming men* or "life gate," gets variably translated into English. The point for him, however, is not the precise terminology, and the "problem" is not one of conveying such terminologically based meaning. Understanding for this translator means fully grasping how the concept relates to a whole system of other concepts that together comprise Chinese medicine, and translation necessarily involves detailed explanation of the "conversation" that emerges out of text-based study:

> It's the whole conversation that comes after that that *explains* what that idea is, that's really the issue. That's why, for me at least, the translation issue is *not* such a big deal. Because I think the real issue is not the individual words we choose, but the fact—whether or not we have the giant concepts down, like the whole, you know.

In invoking the notion of conversation, this translator consciously engages with the interdiscursivity of textuality in Chinese medicine. This perspective informs his choice of translation style, and indeed, in his work he often presents meaning in the context of conversations between him and his various teachers. These conversations involve classical Chinese texts that they interpret together, in conversation with each other, with their past patients, with other contemporary texts they have both read, and with copresent audience members. His translations emerge as a complex, intersubjective, and intertextual arrangement of ideas meant to be read and perused for insights rather than intended as prescriptive guiding of practice. With this conversational style, this translator thus refuses to place much value in getting the individual words right.

Several other translators also highlight the need to refrain from focusing on individual words. They argue for a more "textual" approach, a translation of texts as whole pieces in themselves. Whereas for the first group of translators we looked at, a good translation will access the whole interdiscursive web of classical Chinese knowledge even at the level of individual words and concepts, those scholars who ascribe to the textual view argue that the felt experience of the text as a whole should be the basis for an authentic translation:

> So I think some of the more maybe free-form translation approaches, for lack of a better word … sometimes do a better job in terms of flow and readability, and maintaining the *feel* of the original text.

Here, the scholar emphasizes "flow and readability" in arguing for a more free-form approach to translation, something that does not necessarily "get all the right words":

> And I think sometimes translators make the mistake of getting all the right words, and losing the, the stuff that's in the text that isn't just in the words. What does the text *feel like* to the reader when they read it in English or in Chinese?

This scholar repeats the importance of "feeling" when it comes to authentic translation. In this case, it is a feeling of connection with the text itself rather than with authentic personal experience or authentic understanding of the full dialogic significance of each term used. A textbook, he goes on to say, "should read like a textbook":

> Yeah—I think that there should be— I think that should be an important aspect to translation is that if you're reading—if you're taking a textbook, and translating that textbook into English, the English should read like a textbook, in my opinion. If it's a, a little, you know, *handbook* that somebody wrote that feels very colloquial in the source language? It shouldn't end up feeling like a textbook in English.

For this translator, then, the experience of the text *as a whole* is of primary importance, the source that should be reproduced. And the experience of the whole text, moreover, should be linked to its original purpose as it was written in Chinese. It should convey clinically useful information in a manner that makes that same information available to readers of the text in translation:

> Um, certainly the vast majority of practitioners out in the community with whom I've spoken over the years, could *care less* about this issue. It has no relevance to their practice of Chinese medicine. What they want to know is can you explain that in a way that allows me to use it clinically? Can you represent the concepts from the Chinese in a way that's accurate to what a clinician would get out of them if he or she read that same thing in Chinese?

Over the years, this translator has spoken with a lot of people in the community, and he has heard them when they ask for clinically useful texts, regardless of whether or not they fully convey the deeply interdiscursive nature of each term. Paired with his conviction that "all translation involves loss," this conversation with his students, his readers, leads him to ask "What kind of loss, and how much?" and to answer with his own translations of texts that seek to reproduce whole, clinically applicable books, regardless of terminology.

This section could continue indefinitely, as with each new interview, new perspectives on translation emerged. Some of the most major themes have been described here, however, and together they demonstrate that the act of translation is deeply informed by the way each author perceives and chooses to engage with the interdiscursive web of relationships that comprises practice and textuality in Chinese medicine, including the term debates—how they, as authors, learn to both listen and to speak. It is also, as we have seen, about variable epistemologies of truth and claims about what constitutes the best type of *evidence* for translation. It also happens to be about "creating a medicine," formulating a certain kind of practice and experience through language. In creating this medicine, each author must answer for him or herself what it means to be authentic, to transmit a system of healing originating in a foreign language, and to connect with readers. The diverse answers to these questions, which significantly complicate the simple distinctions made in the debates about standardization and language, give rise to different kinds of translations, different styles of writing and presentation that are themselves reflective of the ongoing interdiscursivity and at the same time can be taken together to understand the way Chinese medicine is variably translated into English. In the next section of this chapter, we thus examine several examples of texts seeking to translate the term *po*.

Inscribing the Soul

In Chinese medicine, the person is comprised of many distinct physical, emotional, mental, and spiritual aspects. These aspects of the self are all intimately connected in relationships that root emotional experience in physical sensations and link specific organs to certain ways of being in the world. There are five components to the "spiritual" or "mental" self, for example, each of which inspires different facets of experience and each of which is intimately tied to a specific organ system, and hence to physical experience. These spirits include the 神 *shen* (spirit), associated with the heart; the 意 *yi* (intellect or reflection), associated with the spleen; the 魄 *po* (corporeal or animal soul), associated with the lungs; the 志 *zhi* (mind or will), associated with the kidneys; and the 魂 *hun* (ethereal soul) associated with the liver. These "five spirits" have proven to be among the most difficult features of Chinese medicine to translate into English clearly. They are the subject of countless attempts, however, as different authors grapple with how best to bridge cultural, historical, philosophical, and linguistic differences in a field that fascinates and draws in the many U.S. students seeking to develop a certain holistic vision of Chinese medicine that heavily favors spiritual and emotional aspects of self, and even in a more limited sense, simply seeks to link mind and body in a coherent frame (Barnes 1998; Van Hoy 2010).

In this section, I closely examine several, though not all, existing translations, interpretations, and explanations of *po*. This is the component of soul, or self, that is most closely linked to the lungs. It is also the aspect of the self that draws "soul" and "body" together in the Chinese medical understanding of movement, intention, and action. Often contrasted with the *hun* or "ethereal soul" of the liver, the meaning of *po* is written into the English language in multiple ways that directly mirror the many complex social, moral, political, and linguistic considerations shaping the translation of Chinese medicine at every level. In the seven examples presented below, I thus show how many of the perspectives introduced in the last section, as well as in the second and third chapters of this book, come to life in specific inscriptions.

Example 1: Reading Po

> **corporeal soul** 魄 *pò*: *synonym: animal soul.* A nonphysical aspect of the human being. *Pò* is the corporeal soul stored by the lung, as distinct from *hún,* the ethereal soul, stored by the liver. *The Magic Pivot* (*líng shū*) states, "That which enters and exists with essence is called the corporeal soul." *The Classified Canon* (*lèi jīng*) states, "The function of the corporeal soul is to enable the body to move and perform its function; pain and itching are felt by it." These descriptions suggest that the corporeal soul is the animating and sensitizing principle that gives humans the ability of movement and physical sensation (Wiseman and Feng 1998: 100)

This first example derives from translators who are well-known to be committed to linguistically precise translations based on specific terms in original Chinese texts. Their goal is faithful mimesis with little to no adaptation of meaning at the level of specific words and concepts. As such, the authors of the *Practical Dictionary* seek to reproduce the intertextual quality of meaning in any Chinese medical term. They do so by embedding straightforward, declarative quotes from classic texts within the body of each definition. The book itself is a thick hard-covered text, totaling over nine hundred pages structured in columns as one finds in a traditional dictionary. There are no illustrations. It is not one of the texts upon which either the national or state board exams are based, although it is the only English language dictionary of Chinese medicine that contains comprehensive definitions alongside translations of specific terms.

The translation style espoused by the authors is reflective of a distinctive and very public philosophy of translation. It is a philosophy that is based on the source-oriented method of Chinese medical translation developed by Nigel Wiseman and colleagues. This translation philosophy, we recall, is based on the belief that "to transmit Chinese medical knowledge to the West, we must translate, not reinvent" (Wiseman 2002b: 22). The social, cultural, and moral justifications for this source-oriented translation philosophy are approached in the last chapter. Here, however, it becomes relevant that the translation philosophy shaping the work is interdiscursive at many levels, including most prominently the level of intertextuality in the original source texts. This is reproduced both in the use of quotes and inclusion of classic text names in *pinyin* with tone marks, as well as the consistent linking of specific translations to Chinese characters. Because Feng is a renowned practitioner as well as scholar, the *Practical Dictionary* is also produced in conversation with clinical practice, although statements are always grounded in the authority of classical texts.

Wiseman and Feng further produce their work in dialogue with the other English-language translations they see available, translations that they very publicly complain do not include proper glossaries, use standard terminology, or translate exactly based on a single authentic Chinese text. In this sense, the final product that they generate is already intertextually linked to other foreign-made products. Finally, the writing of the text is undertaken in conversation with users. In this case, it is a morally situated conversation that asks practitioner and student users to alter their perspective on language in Chinese medicine. As such, it is a critical dialogue, a challenge to readers to shift the basis upon which they approach the source. Through this dialogue, this enactment of translation, Chinese medicine is produced as a historically referenced, textually grounded practice with a definite terminology and a straightforward set of meanings. Translating *po* thus becomes an exercise in precision, including a close examination and direct interpretation of specific historical documents.

Example 2: Approximating Po

> The Corporeal Soul (*Po*) can be defined as "that part of the Soul [as opposed to the Ethereal Soul] which is indissolubly attached to the body and goes down to Earth with it at death." The Corporeal Soul is closely linked to the body and it could be described as the somatic expression of the Soul. As the 'Simple Questions' says in the passage mentioned above, the Corporeal Soul is close to Essence and Qi. The 'Classic of Categories' (1624) says: "The Corporeal Soul moves and accomplishes things and [when it is active] pain and itching can be felt." This passage illustrates just how physical the Corporeal Soul is. It gives us the capacity of sensation, feeling, hearing, and sight (Maciocia 2005: 111).

This translation is quoted from the English-language Chinese medical text titled *The Foundations of Chinese Medicine*. This text, which is one of the two chief texts required in most master's programs in Chinese medicine, is heavily drawn upon in the crafting of state and national board exams, and students must memorize most of the information for those tests as well as for classes. It is a large, heavy book that looks and feels like a textbook, with over twelve hundred glossy pages. Published by Elsevier, it has an officially sanctioned feel to it, complete from paper to font. Aside from the front cover, the section and chapter headings, and some decorative calligraphy, there is little to no Chinese included in the text, although there is a great deal of *pinyin*.

There are many illustrations in the text itself, including many blue highlighted diagrams showing the linear progression of *qi* and other substances throughout the body. There are also many uniform, gender-specific diagrams of bodies. The writing has a very organized, linear feel to it, and the reader is further provided with numerous blue highlighted text boxes that include specific definitions and charts within the margins of each chapter. The book replicates the intertextuality of Chinese texts by commonly quoting classical texts and other scholars of Chinese medicine, although it is never made precisely clear whether these quotes are taken from a specific Chinese translation or are rearranged by the author (the translation of the classic *Lei Jing* or *Classic of Categories* is significantly different from the translation of the same passage included in Wiseman and Feng's text, above). As such, the book is a compilation rather than a direct translation. The author clearly states as much in his preface, where he explains that "I have tried to present the theory of Chinese medicine from Chinese books but I have also occasionally presented my own experience gleaned from 30 years of practice" (Maciocia 2005: vii).

The translations provided by Giovanni Maciocia in *Foundations* are seemingly straightforward and smooth. "For reasons of style," he explains, he capitalizes all Chinese terms and deitalicizes them (Maciocia n.d.: 1). His goal here is to create a "well-written English text" that also reads smoothly (Maciocia n.d.: 1), although it can also be understood as a strategic move in encoding, through capitalization, what Maciocia perceives as a fundamental linguistic difference between Chinese and English. Maciocia's prioritization of reader comfort thus emerges out of a translation philosophy and ideology of language as determinative of worldview that claims that "Chinese philosophical terms are essentially impossible to translate and that, the moment we translate them, we distort them with a world-view that is not Chinese" (Maciocia n.d.: 1–2). He relates the impossibility of translation to the rich heteroglossia informing each Chinese term. Claiming that there is no way to capture this complexity with single terms, he argues against the usefulness of standardized translations and generally aims in his work to provide flexible language depending on context. His text thus emerges as a conversation constructed primarily with his English-speaking audience, in which his own experience along with a loose interpretation of multiple Chinese texts serves as sufficient evidence for translation. Here, Chinese medicine is produced in a dialogue that hinges upon the negotiation of incommensurable differences—between Chinese and English, as well as between theory and practice—in a linear, textbook framework. For translating *po*, this means gathering several historical texts, pairing them with many years of clinical experience, and fashioning a general interpretation of how the *po* "could be" described in English.

Example 3: The Disappearing Po

Interestingly, the other primary textbook required by most master's programs in Chinese medicine in the United States includes neither a detailed description of the mind nor any aspects of the soul. The lack of inclusion of a translation for *po* in this text, however, can actually be seen to be as much of a contribution to the overall interpretation of this term as the other translations included here. This text, a thick hardcover textbook from China, is one of the first translations of Chinese medicine that appeared first in 1987. The preface to the revised edition highlights the international, authoritative status of the text, which has been and continues to be required in most Chinese medical programs in the United States, and is heavily drawn upon in the crafting of state and national board exams. The text is comprehensive, covering basic theory, diagnosis, and treatment, but also going into a great deal more depth with regards to needling methods and the treatment of specific biomedical disease categories such as "dysmenorrhea," "epigastric pain," and "nocturnal enuresis." The text was originally "compiled" under the supervision of the Chinese Ministry of Public Health. Based on *Essentials of Chinese Acupuncture* (a Chinese textbook) and supplemented by "the results of many years of teaching and clinical experience," the foreword states, "*Chinese Acupuncture and Moxibustion* was continually revised, substantiated and perfected" (Chen 2005: foreword, n.p.).

This text, also known as "CAM," is thus clearly a compilation that blurs the line between translation and original. It is an inherently interdiscursive product that liberally incorporates quotes from ancient physicians and classic texts, translating them into English and freely drawing upon biomedical terminology to do so. The first edition, and to a certain extent the revised edition, is poorly edited, with many grammatical errors, typos, and awkward statements. The many illustrations that it includes, however, are extremely realistically rendered and are comprised of detailed colored depictions of specific organs, muscle groups, and "meridians" or channels.

The translation philosophy supporting the production of this text is, like the others we have examined thus far, richly interdiscursive and deeply moral. The foreword talks about "enriching the world's science and culture," a project that we observed in the last chapter is linked to the legitimation of Chinese medicine as a viable mainstream scientific and cultural product. As a zone of encounter or landscape of interpretation in its own right, this textbook indexes the debate, for example, about biomedical terminology and cultural experience. In terms of its intertextuality with classic, source knowledge, it commonly quotes the classics as a legitimation strategy as well as a tactic of cultural representation. The book leverages a scientific, rational interpretation of these classics, however, in translating them into contemporary scientific terms. As a hybrid product emerging out of the ongoing conversation with imagined consumers, the text attempts to produce Chinese medicine as a modern science and technical practice. This is probably the most basic reason for the lack of inclusion of a translation for *po* in CAM. Generally speaking, it is indexical of the Chinese government agenda, in both Communist and contemporary iterations of Chinese medicine, of removing anything that sounds like it is linked to religion in any way. The lung is therefore described in CAM without any reference to the corporeal or animal soul. Instead, it is described as "the hub of vital energy" (Chen 2005: 307) and as the organ responsible for "dominating the *qi* of the whole body" (Chen 2005: 33). It is further described as "a delicate organ … often the first organ to be affected when exogenous pathogenic factors invade the body" (Chen 2005: 307), a scientific analysis of what other texts link to the corporeality of the soul. Interestingly, however, despite the scientific intentions behind CAM's creation, because of the many grammatical errors and inconsistencies it is often perceived by students as a "quaint" representation of how difficult it is to explain Chinese medicine in a linear format (see below).

Example 4: The Science of Po

> Thyroid gland hormones have a relationship to vigor [*po*], since they stimulate oxygen consumption in most cells in the body. They also help regulate fat and carbohydrate metabolism, and are essential for normal growth and development … Thyroxine (T4) and triiodonthyronine (T3) are the main hormones of the thyroid gland … The relationship of thyroid hormones to vigor is through their influence as general regulators of body metabolism, which can increase oxygen consumption, body temperature, pulse rate, systolic blood pressure, and lipolysis, and can decrease serum cholesterol levels. Thyroid hormones control physical vigor and mental alertness, which are major feature of the lung visceral vitality (po) (Kendall 2002: 124–125).

A beautiful hardcover text published by Oxford University Press, *Dao of Chinese Medicine* by Donald Kendall is based on the author's claim that "Chinese medicine is best characterized as a physiological medicine" (2002: 8) based in a solid understanding in ancient China of not only of structural anatomy, but also the vascular system, the endocrine system, and the neurological system, to name a few. The book is not required in most master's programs in Chinese medicine, but it was regularly recommended by at least one instructor in the program where I carried out my research. In it, Kendall charges early

Western mistranslations of Chinese medicine with perpetuating a mischaracterization of Chinese medicine as a mystical or metaphysical, rather than physiological, medicine. This, Kendall argues, happened through a process of "redaction" where incorrect Western translations of original Chinese documents were subsequently adopted by Chinese scholars and physicians. "From the fifteenth century onward, almost all areas of Chinese thought were influenced and revised by Western views and mistranslation … Through the process of redaction, these incorrect terms were adopted by the Chinese to represent the accepted Western terms for the original Chinese" (2002: 3). *Dao of Chinese Medicine* thus emerges out of the quest to describe what the Chinese "really meant," using "universally accepted anatomical and physiological terms" (2002: 9) both to establish "a base line for clinical practice, and also to provide a starting point from which more study can take place" (2002: 9). Kendall thus takes on the task of presenting "the true story—the way or *dao* (道)—of Chinese medicine, so that its basic premise, including its physiological mechanisms, can be viewed in Western terms" (2002: xiii).

Kendall's quest to portray the true story of Chinese medicine is situated, he explains, in "the moral obligation of every practitioner to provide each patient with the latest medical understanding available" (2002: 11). Through a close reading of his text, it becomes clear that the work is also based in the moral commitment to a grand notion of objective truth, including historical and clinical truth, but also pertaining to linguistic accuracy in translation. In this sense, Kendall's aim in this text is nothing short of heroic, a Western scholar and practitioner's attempt to mitigate the effects of hundreds of years of mistranslation and misappropriation on behalf of both Westerners and, subsequently, the Chinese themselves. Throughout the book, then, many ancient texts are quoted simply using bioscientific terminology, with no Chinese included. The translation of *po* as "vigor" with a link to specific thyroid hormones can thus be understood as part of the morally situated conversation with biomedicine, rationality, and science that the text as a whole seeks to present.

Examples 5–7: Putting the Poetry Back in Po

Example 5

Po is the portion of a person's Spirit that is absolutely dependent on the person's physical life … The Po is about momentary reactions; unlike the other Spirits … it is utterly tied to time and space. Po is the reactivity or animation of a person, hence the alternative translation Animal Soul (Kaptchuk 2000: 64).

Example 6

The *po* consists of the seven emotions (fear, anxiety, anger, joy, sorrow, worry, and grief) which are the primal urges that facilitate the grasping of life. As an earth-

> bound spirit, I think of the *po* as relating to gravity, a force that draws things in toward the center of our being and holds them there. The function of the *po* is to contact what is of essential worth, receive it into (lungs), and retain it within (large intestine) while returning the *yin* mundane influences back to the earth from whence they came ... The *po* turns the nourishing *yang* (sunlight) of later heaven, which is contained in air and captured by all that grows, into the body. Upon death the *po* becomes fertilizer, returning to earth in a way that empowers new growth (Jarrett 1998: 260).

> *Example 7*
> The po are the animating agents of vital life processes that take place beyond our conscious awareness and control. They are closely related to the autonomic nervous system, the sensory receptors ... [The *po*] can be correlated with more primitive aspects of the brain such as the limbic system and cerebellum ... The po are the buried light of spirit. They are the complexes, psychosomatic symptoms, emotional blocks and intuitive knowing that lock in psychic energy that can be later unraveled and used for our psychological development. The treasures of our embodied soul hide in these crystallized structures, the tangled psychic knots of consciousness ... The po are our embodied knowing, our animal wit, our street smarts, the part of us that can sniff out what's right or wrong, good or bad, safe or unsafe (Dechar 2006: 238–239).

Example 5 emerges from the second edition of a more compact paperback book, elegantly illustrated and produced in a comfortable, contemporary font. Like the first text introduced in this section, it is written as an introduction to the basic concepts of Chinese medicine, covering everything from Chinese medical anatomy to diagnosis to treatment. The target audience includes English-speaking students of Chinese medicine, but it also includes other, more public audiences—patients and everyday interested readers. And so in contrast to the first text, it also includes chapters on the art and philosophy of Chinese medicine, with poetic discussions of the nature of truth and the role of spirituality in treatment. For this reason, this text is often recommended to students when they first begin their Chinese medical studies, even prior to their first class. It is extremely popular and has already come out in a second edition, complete with a foreword by holistic health guru Andrew Weil. It is not, however, required by many schools, nor is it used in the development of national or state board exams.

The writing in this text is poetic, even beautiful. It is a flowing style of writing that is interspersed with some Chinese characters and some *pinyin* transliterations, as well as many literal illustrations of various parts of the human body with one or more acupuncture channels depicted along the isolated chest or leg. Like in *Foundations*, the Chinese terms here are capitalized, with translations explained in the text itself rather than in footnotes, although there are also extensive, intertextual footnotes included at the end of each chapter, in much smaller font. It is not a direct translation of any single Chinese text, emerging more as a hybrid built, as the author explains it, out of years of studying Chinese classic texts, seeing patients in hospitals and clinics, and working with academicians at Harvard. It has emerged, he explains in his introduction, as a result of personal encounters as well as scholarly encounters with science, medical history, and anthropology. It has also developed, he writes, in interactions with patients who "have demanded that my practice of Chinese medicine embody authenticity and relevance" (Kaptchuk 2000: xxiv). In this sense, Kaptchuk's *The Web That Has No Weaver: Understanding Chinese Medicine* is a text that is deeply interdiscursive at many levels: social, cultural, textual, personal. The final result emerges out of this interdiscursivity as a decidedly practical and moral project that seeks to provide an authentic and "relevant" medical guidebook, rather than an academic treatise that attempts to overtly engage with the inherent intertextuality of Chinese medicine. He explains:

> I have grown acutely aware that East Asian medicine is a huge ocean of texts and interpretations. Any assertion is automatically a complex problematic and an opportunity for contending understandings. My hermeneutic tendency would have liked to pursue the paradoxical knowledge produced by irreducible uncertainty. For this edition, this tendency was overruled (or at least sometimes just moved to a footnote.) I wanted this *Web*, like its predecessor, to continue being an introduction to a coherent and *radically distinct* approach toward medicine. *I want it to ultimately embody hope.* Patients need treatment. Practitioners need strategies. Many intellectual problems have been put aside. In the choice between an analytic deconstructionism and provocative narrative, I have adopted the perspective that healing must embody an art with a compelling and even poetic message (Kaptchuck 2000: xxv–xxvi, italics mine).

For Ted Kaptchuk, then, text creation is an act of *hope*. It is a social action geared toward the development of clear strategies rather than the "hermeneutic" teasing out of "intellectual problems." Its authenticity derives from clinical interactions that demand a "compelling and even poetic message." In this sense, the text is a conversation in which Kaptchuk engages his readers by inviting them into a "distinct" world of Chinese medicine, a different ethos of body, illness, and healing. Rather than challenging readers to learn about the historically situated practice of Chinese medicine, it takes them on a narrative journey that produces Chinese medicine as a complementary and alternative medical practice with holistic techniques and a foundation in poetry. In this context, *po* becomes a part of the capital-S Spirit. It is further tied to phenomenological experience in the form of "momentary reactions" that Kaptchuk likens to an aspect of self that he anticipates Western readers will understand more clearly as their "Animal Soul."

The second explanation of *po*, which invokes the notion of the *po* as a central force drawing the outside world into the core of a person, comes from a thick, elegant text entitled *Nourishing Destiny: The Inner Tradition of Chinese Medicine*. It is written, like many of the other texts in this section, as an introductory view on many of the basic theories of Chinese medicine, including *yin-yang*, *qi*, and the five phases. In contrast to some of the other texts included here, however, this book has a clear and overarching spiritual message. In each section, different Chinese concepts are related to the quest of "nourishing destiny," fulfilling individual selfhood, and the "inner tradition" of Chinese medicine. In the author's words, "The term 'inner tradition' refers to the practice of Chinese medicine in a way that places primary emphasis on the use of medicine as a tool to aid spiritual evolution … and explicitly serves as an extension of the practitioner's own spiritual quest and path" (Jarrett 1998: xxii). The text is thus very much tied to the spiritually framed task of a particular American population seeking a certain kind of individual and societal evolution through experientially resonant practice. This is very much in alignment with the notion of hope and transformation supported in example 5. Almost half of the last part of the book thus contains case studies from contemporary American contexts, discussing them in terms of the authors own individual perspectives and showing the application of the inner tradition for various kinds of distress.

Although it is not immediately readable from the translation of *po*, the book is deeply intertextual, quoting many classic Chinese texts and classic Chinese philosophers (or English translations of such material) as well as contemporary American spiritual, scientific, and philosophical texts. As such, it stands as a compilation, an original hybrid comprised of disparate pieces arranged together based on the clinical, cultural, and spiritual experiences of the author in conjunction with the scholarly pursuit of certain strands of Chinese history and philosophy, particularly Daoist alchemical texts, as well as a clearly referenced background in neuroscience. The main text portions of the book contain some, mostly single, Chinese characters, and there are many *pinyin* terms. Key characters, some written in large calligraphy and placed at the beginnings of section headings, are presented with etymological explanations clearly favoring a spiritual interpretation. In the section heading preceding the excerpt above, for example, the character for *po* is etymologically examined as containing the character for "white" (*bai*) on the left and the character for "earthbound spirits" (*gui*) on the right. "White is the color of metal," Jarrett explains, "and the *po* is the *shen* associated with the lungs" (1998: 259). Jarrett provides some further explanation of this etymology by explaining that the color white is included as a representation of "the color of bones that lie curried within the earth" (1998: 260). "Upon death," he continues, "the *po* descends through the anus and returns to earth" (1998: 260).

Besides characters, there are drawings of cosmic phenomenon such as holographic images and laser light waves. It is not a required text, nor is it included on the state or national tests, but especially because of its firm commitment to a spiritual interpretation of Chinese medicine, it is extremely popular with students and is often referenced in the classroom. Formed with a very explicit "translation philosophy," this book is written in a nonlinear format that seeks to reproduce the nonlinearity of classical Chinese. The significance of the information in the text is meant, Jarrett explains, to "only emerge in context once the entire book has been read" (Jarrett 1998: xi). Translations are liberal, with ultimate authority resting not with some external measure of accuracy but instead with the author's own experience. A fairly well-known figure, this particular author's experience is also heavily invested in what he terms, in an e-mail sent out to the educational community in 2008, the creation of a "new medicine for a new humanity." In this new medicine, Jarrett claims, there will be no more time-consuming "processing" as part of healing. Emerging as a grand-scale shift in consciousness, healing will be instant and spontaneous, as the authentic Self comes online: "From this perspective any modality that requires 'process' is seen as strengthening the presence of the disease by reinforcing a dysfunctional relationship to time, thought, and feeling." With this overarching goal, it is not surprising that translation should likewise require little technical process, emerging instead as a conversation with purposely selective cultural experience. *Po* here becomes a sense of primal, emotional urgency that simultaneously contains the seed for transformation, reempowerment, and self-growth.

The final example of a translation for *po* as "agents of vital life processes that take place beyond our conscious awareness and control" derives from another spiritually oriented text created explicitly in order to facilitate "an efficient technology for psychospiritual transformation" (Dechar 2006: xix). It is thus aptly titled *Five Spirits: Alchemical Acupuncture for Psychological and Spiritual Healing*. An elegantly crafted paperback, *Five Spirits* weaves together images of Daoist sages sitting upon mountaintops in ancient China with authoritative explanations of Chinese culture, Chinese medicine, and Chinese language. It is a story of the author's personal journey at the same time as it is a manifesto for a new model of nonlinear consciousness and healing. The overarching goal of the book, Dechar explains, is to use Chinese medicine "as a springboard to a new and more efficient system of emotional, psychosomatic, and psychospiritual healing" (2006: xv).

Using an etymological style of translation similar to that examined in example 6, Dechar thus includes many Chinese characters, displayed in calligraphy outside of the main narrative text. The emphasis here is on the translation of single terms rather than complete texts or even full sentences and phrases. The author explains this by saying that "[f]rom my own experience, the original characters provide the key to understanding ancient Chinese concepts and no translation can compare to studying the ancient graphics themselves" (Dechar 2006: xvi). For each extensive etymological explanation of specific Chinese characters, she divulges her sources as consisting of Chinese etymological dictionaries, a popular software program, and study of the recorded talks of scholars in the field. "I have amplified my interpretation of the characters," Dechar adds, "through insights gleaned from studies of Buddhist and Taoist philosophy, archetypal psychology, and the symbolic language of dreams and the collective unconscious" (2006: xvi). In this sense, Dechar identifies the evidence for her translations as emerging directly out of a hybrid, multivalent conversation with several differentially positioned authorities.

Like several of the examples included in this chapter, *Five Spirits* is not a required text for state or national exams. It is a popular text amongst Westerners desperately craving a more psychospiritual explanation of Chinese medicine, however, and so it is included here as an example of how certain translations can be simultaneously biomedical and psychological, spiritual, and poetic and can be read as a direct index of these enduring, wildly interdiscursive conversations. Dechar's description of the *po* as related to the autonomic nervous system, the limbic system, and the cerebellum, for example, indexes her desire to create a translation that can speak comfortably to biomedical framings of the body. In calling the *po* "the buried light of spirit," however, Dechar further indexes her position as an author who understands the intricate process of psychological development from a spiritual, emotional perspective that also incorporates Chinese medicine. The *po* thus become "tangled knots of psychic consciousness" at the same time as they retain the "primitive" or "intuitive" animal awareness of right and wrong. Deeply physical, and deeply moral, the *po* are translated here at the intersection of multiple, ongoing conversations with biomedicine, New Age spirituality, and humanistic psychology.

Discussion and Conclusion

That the library of texts in Chinese medicine is richly interdiscursive is indisputable. In this chapter, I have shown that this inherent interdiscursivity challenges different translators to construct meaningful texts that somehow capture a particular slice of this "mangle of practice" (Pickering 1995). I have shown that the way this emerges is far from arbitrary. Data from both sections of this chapter show that this project is heavily mediated by ideologies of authenticity, morality, hope, language, and translation, as well as through each author's engagement in conversations with real and imagined audiences. Visions of humanity, philosophy, and poetry play a role, informing how each inscription takes shape. The desire to shape practice, to influence minds, to contribute to the advancement of science or the evolution of consciousness, all of these things are very real factors shaping the choices that translators make and the particular pieces of the conversation that they highlight with their texts. *Po* thus becomes something scientific or something spiritual—or nothing at all—depending on where you look. In this sense, textuality in Chinese medicine is a living practice in which past, present, and future authors carry on meaningful dialogues with their students, their patients, and their colleagues in biomedicine, psychology, and the New Age.

Understanding textuality and translation as living practices, themselves zones of encounter with far-reaching implications, compels a series of questions related to the social politics of translation in Chinese medicine briefly examined in the last chapter. Who or what, we might ask, is being conquered in each form of translation? What is lost, for example, when a pocket-sized handbook becomes a hardback scholarly text in translation? Where does the original lie in the stream of interdiscursivity that is textuality in Chinese medicine? If we agree that in this constant recitation and strategic quoting of past scholars, the original "melts away," does it then become okay to simply translate only what seems to matter in the moment? Similarly, at what point should an individual have the right to engage in authoritative translation? What is the validity of his or her experience in translating? Is it only the experience of Chinese practitioners that counts? When, in other words, is a translation authentic and how does hybridity complicate this authenticity?

These are all complex questions, and while I do not purport to try to answer them definitively here, I am particularly interested in examining what an anthropological appreciation of interdiscursivity and intertextuality can contribute to their emerging answers. I am therefore interested in the "worldly" impact of the multiple translations that are created in the everyday lives of users—how they learn to listen in situations where multiple translation live together. The texts we are speaking about, after all, are crafted with the intention of being used (and indeed are used) in both educational and clinical contexts.

As a practice, then, the living nature of textuality in Chinese medicine only begins with the way the texts are written. As mentioned above, it continues in the social life of the texts. The products all live together, not singly or apart from one another. In the context of the school, the texts are discussed on a daily basis. As I show in the next chapters, the translations that they offer are analyzed and compared vis-à-vis the authority and experience of particular teachers, as well as the embodied experiences of individual students. In listening to lectures, and reading the texts themselves, the students become involved with the books.

This involvement, Sterponi explains "is not so much an internalization of the text as an interaction with it" (2004: 11). In their comments to me over the course of two to three years, students consistently emphasized the very personal nature of the relationship they form with their books and, by extension, with certain authors. In discussing the sterile, scientific style of Maciocia, for example, Julia explains that "I'm just not feeling the medicine from Maciocia." Another student, Oren, compares Maciocia's approach to the style in CAM. "I feel like Maciocia's raping me," he says emphatically, "whereas CAM is seducing me." CAM feels like more of an "old-soul" book says Sarah, despite the tendency for CAM to use more scientific jargon to translate Chinese medicine. It's the feel of the book, these students explain, including the smell and texture of the pages. None of them argue that Maciocia's style is not more straightforward, however, and as they proceed through the program their favoring of CAM wanes considerably. Treavor thus describes Maciocia as "knowing how to feed [the concepts] to an English speaker." Because of this, he is inclined to find Maciocia "more credible." But, because "it's coming from the horse's mouth," he is also inclined to find CAM more reliable. "They both have their merits," he continues. "And ultimately, because I'm the one who's going to be in charge of my own practice, I just need to learn what I can learn from both of them, and incorporate them into my own understanding, as much of it as I can in a way that doesn't cause me to have brain hemorrhage." From this vantage point, texts in Chinese medicine are "indeterminate" (Sterponi 2004, 2007) until picked up and read, interpreted and experienced in connection with other texts, as well as clinical experience and classroom interaction.

In combination with the view of translation as social action, this perspective further questions the traditional boundaries separating text from nontext, as "extratextual" factors permeate the creation and the interpretation of texts along sometimes unexpected lines (Hanks 1989). The surface use of scientific lingo in CAM, for example, is not necessarily experienced as more modern or Westernized by students craving a more traditional interaction. In this case, the consumption of the information in the texts is contingent upon a great many factors, including first and foremost the sensual engagement with the book itself. The translations enacted within each book, moreover, are necessarily filtered through this deeply embodied and profoundly social engagement. What I venture to suggest in this study is that, as students and teachers in the context of Chinese medical school interact with and become involved with their texts, they simultaneously participate in the ongoing set of conversations by which Chinese medicine is collaboratively translated. Whether we are talking about *po* or any other concept, the living translation of Chinese medicine is enacted in all of these conversations. In the next chapter I offer a close examination of how students and teachers engage with translation in texts and across texts in the context of the school.

CHAPTER

4

Interaction in the Living Translation of Chinese Medicine

Lemme tell ya that this whole issue of nomenclature in Chinese medicine just sucks. It really, really sucks. Translation sucks. Comparative nomenclature from book to book sucks. I mean tell me, does this not suck? It makes our job so much harder, and the reason for you guys it makes it so much harder is because you have textbooks that the state board relies on to write exams, and very often the nomenclature in those textbooks is misleading and not clinically relevant. So you know, bad for you, you gotta learn things the wrong way, and then you've got to apply them clinically in a completely different way. So I'm gonna try with this thready pulse to actually give you both and give you the explanation of why what's written in the book isn't necessarily as clinically accurate as it should be, ok?

—Barbara, instructor in first-year Diagnosis class

In the last chapter, I demonstrate that textuality in Chinese medicine is a richly interdiscursive and lively process, a mode of social action (Hanks 1989) that is ongoing as authors create texts as conversations with past, present, and future practice. I also introduced the notion of textual indeterminacy that resides in the various ways in which students, as the primary users of texts, become involved with their books (Sterponi 2004, 2007). Such involvement unfolds as a deeply personal, social interaction with the language of the texts, a learning how to listen where meaning emerges in concert with contact with texts as objects of consumption. In this sense, interpretations of texts are achieved in a "dialectic" that can best be conceived as carrying on the set of conversations that together comprise living translation. "Only through [the interpreter] are the written marks changed back into meaning," writes Gadamer (2004 [1975]: 389):

> One intends to *understand the text itself.* But this means that the interpreter's own thoughts too have gone into re-awakening the text's meaning. In this the interpreter's own horizon is decisive, yet not as a personal standpoint that he maintains or

> enforces, but more as an opinion and a possibility that one brings into play and puts at risk, and that helps one truly to make one's own what the text says (Gadamer 2004 [1975]: 390).

While Gadamer here is referring to the reading of texts, his analysis also pertains when there is an outside interpreter helping the reader make sense of the material. In Agha's words, "[T]he artifacts that disseminate these normative discourses [dictionaries, handbooks] have a social life only through the mediation of speech chains linking persons to each other" (2007: 129). In a classroom context, for example, where texts are inevitably invoked and reinterpreted constantly, lives the opportunity to witness the community coming to an understanding of meaning through talk about texts (see Pritzker 2012d). In this sense, although translations are apparently laid down in certain texts, their "life" in the community is only awakened through interpretive interaction, especially in interaction about language.

In this chapter, I show how the plurality of translations in available Chinese medical texts is approached in the classroom and how teachers and students engage with the multiple translations in such a way as to eventually come to a working understanding of the material in English. So even though all instruction in this U.S. school takes place in English, the presence of "translation talk" is constant. Students and teachers are continuously reminding each other that "this medicine" originates in a foreign land, with foreign customs and a foreign language, and that it must be translated into English and into an American context. Discussions regarding which translations are better or more accurate (or even easier to understand)—and what other teachers or mentors may have said about a text or term—are thus a part of everyday interaction in this school (see Bauman 2004). This is a situation that provides an excellent opportunity to observe translation in Chinese medicine as a lived event involving both textual artifacts and oral transmission. Because multiple participants contribute to the indeterminate conversation, however, these necessary translations become subject to varying strategies, dispositions, and practices accomplished through interaction in the school environment, within texts, in the classroom, and beyond. Much more beyond "just" translation is accomplished in such interactions. Translation in Chinese medicine is also a performance, an opportunity to interactively demonstrate one's linguistic, cultural, or scholarly expertise, to build a case for interpreting evidence in specific ways, and to demonstrate (and sometimes to learn) what language is and what language does. It is also, I suggest, an occasion to learn about how to *practice* Chinese medicine—how to make clinical choices regarding diagnosis and treatment based on a certain understanding of language. Living translation here is enacted in a constant stream of interaction and collaborative social action, an engaged human process of interpretation of meaning across linguistic and cultural boundaries through conversation.

In the taxonomy of living translation, this chapter thus describes the "interaction" phase of the process. As in other phases of living translation, interaction is always mediated by the other phases—inscription, embodied experience, and practice—as well as the multiple historical, institutional, moral, and material frameworks that permeate the field. The chapter is broken up into four sections. The first and second sections provide further introduction and background information on interaction, authority, and evidentiality strategies in the enactment of translation in the Chinese medical classroom. The third and fourth sections offer ethnographic examples of the translation of single terms *qi* and *yin*. Both of these ethnographic sections include several instances showing students taking up the invitation to participate in translation, formulating their own morally situated and culturally grounded strategies as classroom conversations extend into their own self-positioning in the field. I conclude by discussing the process of translation-through-interaction as an ongoing hermeneutic endeavor that results in the socially situated interpretation of language in Chinese medicine in the United States. It is also, as I show below, a social process of (1) establishing authority, (2) creating an evidential basis for decision-making in practice, and (3) articulating, sharing, and resisting various ideologies of language.

Living Translation in Interaction

The view of living translation as interactive is grounded in a sociolinguistic and anthropological understanding of interaction and co-construction as the social process by which meaning is jointly formulated. This section discusses this background in more detail. As Ochs and Jacoby explain:

> We refer to co-construction as *the joint creation of a form, interpretation, stance, action, activity, identity, institution, skill, ideology, emotion, or other culturally meaningful reality.* The *co-* prefix in *co-construction* is intended to cover a range of interactional processes, including collaboration, cooperation, and coordination (Ochs and Jacoby 1995: 171, italics in original).

Meaning here is produced in interaction. In examining what this might mean for translation, Wadensjö (1998) calls attention to the limitations of the source-target "conduit model" in apprehending the complexity of the translation process:

> Interpreters are thought of, and think of themselves, as conveyers of others' words and utterances. The interpreter as channel through which prepared messages go back and forth is a model that is perfectly in line with the norm of non-involvement. The conduit model is *monological* ... The *dialogical* model, in contrast, implies that

the meaning conveyed in and by talk is partly a joint product (Wadensjö 1998: 8, italics in original).

Wadensjö's perspective on translation thus challenges the traditional binary distinction of source and target, arguing that the result is achieved literally in the conversation. By focusing on interpretation, rather than written translation, Wadensjö especially highlights the real-time interactive unfolding of translation. Also discussing oral translation, Michael Cronin similarly suggests an increased involvement of engaged participants, "One could argue that the moment of translation marks a shift from an encounter scene as a site of consumption to a site of interaction. Through the newfound ability to communicate via translation, "the traveler is no longer an observer but part of what is being observed" (Cronin 2002: 60). In this sense, interpretive practices in the translation of Chinese medicine in spoken interaction become part of what is being translated, especially intralingually, but also interlingually and intersemiotically as well.

In concert with a language socialization perspective, which holds that "the child or the novice (in the case of older individuals) is not a passive recipient of sociocultural knowledge but rather an active contributor to the meaning and outcome of interactions with other members of a social group" (Schieffelin and Ochs 1986: 165), this view on translation allows us to consider teachers and students who participate in translation talk as participants in the overall process by which Chinese medicine is collaboratively translated into English. It also shifts the understanding of "context" in the translation of Chinese medicine from an outside influence or ideology *shaping* translation to an *emergent* variable that includes everyday participants. As Goodwin and Duranti discuss, "instead of viewing context as a set of variables that statically surrounds strips of talk, context and talk are now argued to stand in a mutually reflexive relationship to each other" (1992: 31). Similar to the sociocultural understanding of translation as ongoing and emergent in interactions over time, this view asks us to go further in tracing participation in interaction by conducting fine-grained analyses of everyday talk.

The idea of participation here is critical for understanding how translation emerges in interaction in the current research context. Seeing students in this study as participants in translation is, first and foremost, grounded in the theoretical approaches of co-construction, language socialization, and translation studies. However, the situation in the school is also unique in that the students understand themselves as participants in shaping the future of Chinese medicine in the United States. Like the participants in Flesch's study, for example, who conceived "of themselves as pioneers, visionaries, revolutionaries on the cusp of dramatic change in American society" (2010: 237), the students in the present study consider themselves active participants in the translation of

Chinese medicine. This participation, we will see, is supported by talk about translation in school. Students and teachers alike thus learn, through interaction, that "doing translation" is a key part of the requirement for becoming a successful and effective practitioner, as well as for the successful transmission of Chinese medicine in the United States. In this sense, translation talk in Chinese medicine is a social tool at the same time as it unfolds as a social process that hinges not only upon language, but also what people are accomplishing with language when they engage in translation practices.

Authority, Evidence, and Ideologies of Language in the Chinese Medical Classroom

In a field like Chinese medicine, where there is so much unevenness with regard to participants' knowledge of Chinese language, culture, and literature, it is useful to keep in mind that, even though a co-constructive perspective acknowledges that "there is a distributed responsibility among interlocutors for the creation of sequential coherence, identities, meanings, and events" (Ochs and Jacoby 1995: 177), this does not necessarily erase the complex relations of power that are perpetuated in selective acts of translation:

> Co-construction certainly does not mean that participants play identical interactional roles or that through interaction asymmetrical social relations fall away into an egalitarian utopia (Ochs and Jacoby 1995: 178).

In the context of the school, where the students get only one quarter of Chinese medical language and only a few of the teachers speak or write Chinese fluently, the fact that teachers serve as the first primary interpreters of texts for students provides an ideal venue to examine the social politics of translation in Chinese medicine. This section approaches the dynamics of this involvement.

Interpreters are traditionally seen as taking part "in situations where they have a unique opportunity to understand everything said and therefore a unique position from which to exercise a certain control" (Wadensjö 1998: 105). This power of the interpreter, Anderson explains, is rooted in the control of "scarce resources" (1976: 218, as cited in Cronin 2002). In Chinese medicine, however, the resources are not so much scarce as they are plural. With multiple original sources, multiple translated sources, and multiple perspectives on experience and historical significance, translation talk in Chinese medicine reflects multiple ideologies jointly produced in interactions that themselves provide a ground for establishing social authority and social action.

Toury writes that "'Translatorship' amounts first and foremost to being able to *play a social role*, i.e., to fulfill a function allotted by a community" (2000

[1978]: 198, italics in original). Aside from simple teaching strategies, these roles often relate to participants' need to establish legitimacy as players in the complex field of countless Chinese texts and multiple English translations (see Fox 2001). Translation talk in this sense is used as a platform for positioning oneself in relation to "original" or "traditional" Chinese knowledge, whether or not one speaks Chinese. Translation talk and the evidence used to support it can thus be understood as a form of social and discursive deixis (Clift 2006) in which participants epistemically position themselves with regards to information originating in a different language and time. In a field in which teachers have varying degrees of skill in both Chinese and English, it is also a major way in which participants interactively establish the authority to report on the validity of certain translations and interpretations and thus to participate in translation in the first place (see Duranti 1993; Fox 2001; Hill and Irvine 1993; Shuman 1993).

As with other scenarios in which uncertainty prevails (Pomerantz 1984), and like translators themselves, teachers use different kinds of evidence to support their claims about various ways to translate Chinese medical concepts, and in so doing they demonstrate what *counts* as evidence in a clinical sense as well. After lodging the complaint about translation quoted in the opening of this chapter, for example, Barbara uses an "evidentiality strategy" (Aikhenvald 2004) that privileges clinical experience over "misleading" texts to translate the Chinese term otherwise understood as a "thready" pulse. "So I'm gonna try with this thready pulse to actually give you both [clinical definitions and translations in texts] and give you the explanation of why what's written in the book isn't necessarily as clinically accurate as it should be," Barbara says, foregrounding her presentation of different types of evidence. Although English does not have grammaticalized evidentials, specific grammatical forms that convey the "ways in which the information was acquired" (Aikhenvald 2004: 3) such as in languages like Hopi, where information about how the speaker knows what he or she knows (through hearsay, through direct observation, etc.) is encoded grammatically in the sentence, English speakers do draw upon different strategies, sometimes more or less overt, for conveying how we know what we know, whether it is through inference, direct observation, or felt experience. In the current example, Barbara argues against a certain translation based on what she has seen in the clinic. In this sense, she draws upon an evidentiality strategy that privileges experience over and above the translated text to challenge the translation of the Chinese term. In other cases, teachers draw upon evidentiality strategies that privilege canonical textuality as the foundation for correct translations. Teachers differ, however, as to which texts they draw upon as authorities in such cases—English scholarly texts, original Chinese textbooks, Chinese classics, or scientific interpretations of classics. Still other participants locate evidence for certain translations in cultural or aesthetic experience, where everyday involvement in cultural contexts serves as the ultimate evidential basis for action. Different participants, moreover, draw upon different strategies at different times. Such decisions are very much mediated by the historical, institutional, and moral forces at work in shaping any specific interaction.

Finally, translation talk in Chinese medicine often occurs in relation to the distinct ideologies of language and translation discussed in chapter 2, variably drawing upon notions of language as referential, language as unimportant in comparison with divine Truth (located in the body), language as the outward expression of thought, language as cultural capital, language as abstraction, or language as a tool—for accessing foreign knowledge, for empowerment, or for deciphering classics by introducing us to the vast network of interconnected meanings (Bakhtin 1981, 1986). In this sense, the arguments that teachers and students make about translation and how to interpret language in Chinese medicine in moments of translation talk are tied to variable notions of authenticity, truth, the purpose of healing, and the goal of translation. For teachers, evidentiality strategies are further informed by the way they understand their roles in relation to their students, and by the ways in which they interpret texts and explain translations to them. It is in translation talk, in other words, where we can witness the ways in which multiple ideologies of language and translation mediate the enactment of translation as a collaborative act. It is also in translation talk where we begin to see the ways in which ideologies of language and translation shift over time and often provide a basis for moments of socialization where the foundations for future clinical action are laid out.

Translation in Interaction I: Rendering *Qi*

In the following set of examples, I show the ways in which, through dialogue about how to translate the term *qi,* teachers and students collaboratively achieve multiple translations of this foundational Chinese medical term in English. In previous chapters, this term has come up multiple times. This is because, for English speakers, *qi* is perhaps the most widely recognized Chinese medical word. Translated variously as "energy," "life force," and "finest matter influences," *qi* is a complex, physically real term that every student, teacher, and translator encounters early in their efforts to learn, explain, translate, or practice Chinese medicine. It is often the first term used to justify the moral position that Chinese medicine is primarily an intuitive, embodied practice. It is also brought up as an example of the arbitrariness of language, or the impossibility of translation. In this section, however, I want to shift the focus to look at how *qi* does get translated, through interaction, even when it does not. In other words, I want to look at the ways in which interaction serves as the collaborative ground for meaning-making in regards to this complex term.

In text-based translation, it is generally accepted that each author must set forth his or her own guidelines for translating and explaining *qi* in English. In other words, authors are responsible for establishing their own evidence to defend their strategy for translating this basic term, and often such strategies are closely linked to the particular author's overall ideologies of language, translation, and cultural difference. For example, *qi* is often held up as the gold standard evidence that Chinese medicine is fundamentally different than biomedicine. In Ted Kaptchuk's *Web That Has No Weaver,* he thus explains that "no one English word or phrase can adequately capture Qi's meaning" (2000: 43). Even as this description invokes an ideology of incommensurability, however, he goes on to explain *qi,* with the qualification that any English definition falls short of capturing the depth of this core Chinese concept, as "a kind of matter on the verge of becoming energy, or energy at the point of materializing" (2000: 43). Maciocia echoes the sentiment that *qi* is hard to translate, explaining that "the reason it is so difficult to translate the word 'Qi' correctly lies precisely in the versatile nature whereby *qi* can assume different manifestations and be different things in different situations" (2005: 41). Maciocia, like Kaptchuk, therefore favors leaving it untranslated. He does, however, offer several English language explanations of *qi,* including one that explains it as "the very basis of the universe's infinite manifestations of life" (Maciocia 2005: 42). Both Kaptchuk and Maciocia capitalize the term as "Qi" (no italics). In doing so, they strategically deploy an orthographic resource (capitalization) to mark Chinese concepts as different from Western ones. Rochat de la Vallée also offers a detailed explanation for the many meanings of *qi* in Chinese, saying that "there can be a state of undifferentiated totality in which everything is qi" and that "it can be the life-giving principle, original qi, or the components of the constituent agent of all which exists" (2006: 8). She continues to explain that *qi* can be "life force and activity in any organism or phenomenon, the vigor of motion, energy, the animating forces of the universe" or that it can also mean tangible things like "breath, steam, gas or vapour." (2006: 8). All of these meanings, she suggests, are observable within the traditional Chinese character for *qi* (氣), a pictograph of steam rising from rice as it cooks.

With so many aspects and potentialities, *qi* is understandably a difficult concept to translate and explain. Most authors therefore borrow the *pinyin* term *qi,* usually without italicization. As it becomes clear in their descriptions, however, this borrowing does not free them from the requirement of explaining *qi* in English, using indexically grounded ways of speaking to describe the many aspects of this illusive and multifaceted expression. Discussion about how to translate this basic Chinese medical term thus forms a major foundation upon which the texts are built, with each author participating in the translation process and positioning themselves with regards to the original by offering a slightly different interpretation.

Discussion of *qi* is no different in the context of classroom dialogue. In this setting, teachers must also put forth a strategy or strategies for translating *qi*, and in so doing they initiate students into the contingency of translation in Chinese medicine from day one of their education. By showing students how to engage with translation in Chinese medicine, teachers also interactively accomplish the grounds for their own authority to participate in the interpretation process and show students that participation involves positioning oneself with regards to available sources.

Let's Talk about Qi

The first example takes place on the second day of the students' first quarter. Their teacher, Carter, is giving a lecture on the basic elements of the body. Sparked by a question-response sequence initiated by Carter, this leads to a discussion of how to translate the term *qi*. The dialogic sequence begins with a question:

> Carter: [L]et's talk about *qi*. Because that's something that we talk about a lot. So (1.8) even though we'll go into greater detail later (.) let's have a general, ah, idea about it right now=generally translated as (.) anybody?

By prompting the students' participation, Carter is overtly involving them in the conversation. From the start, then, students are brought into the discussion of translation as participants, albeit unequal ones in terms of their authority to contribute to the actual translation of *qi* in this context. Their responses, called out simultaneously, include two common translations: "energy" and "life force." Carter uses these responses as a launching off point to teach them about translation and some of the ways it is commonly handled:

> Carter: Life force, or energy, that's pretty typical, ah, translation (1.8) um (4.5) and that's a tricky one (.), ah, to translate. So a lot of people don't bother translating it, actually. That's why you see *qi* written everywhere, and not life force or energy.

Here, Carter acknowledges that both *life force* and *energy* are "typical" translations, at once offering an assessment of the students' translations, asserting the right to assess their responses, and tacitly indexing his expert knowledge of all available translations (see Heritage and Raymond 2005). Following this, he explains that, although these particular translations are common, the term is actually "a tricky one to translate." Because of this trickiness, he continues, a lot of "people" (i.e., experts) do not "bother" to translate it. With this juxtaposition of typical or common translations with the more expert practice of not translating the term at all, Carter initiates students into an expert world in which translation is no longer straightforward or easy. In fact, in this world, to be a competent translator or practitioner of Chinese medicine, one does not even necessarily need to find English terms for key words, although one must still be versed in various ways of speaking about the concept for the purpose of explanation. This initiation also serves as the grounds for Carter's further demonstration of his own evidential strategy for both translating and teaching translation, a strategy that draws upon multiple English-language scholarly authorities in order to demonstrate the complexities of translation as well as to ultimately translate the term using multiple explanations. He also uses it as an opportunity to teach his students that every time they use an English term to talk about something in Chinese medicine, they are participating in translation:

> Carter: Um (.) the reason is that *qi* is considered not just to be, ah (.) energy=ah (.) but also to have material, ah, a material aspect, material components. And the translation as energy sort of con-conceals that (0.8) It doesn't (1.2) shed light on that. Um (1.8)

In this portion of the interaction, despite his earlier comment that many experts do not translate the term at all, Carter is responding to the students' use of the term "energy" to translate *qi*. By saying that this translation conceals the material aspects of the phenomenon that "are considered" to exist, Carter again invokes an authoritative understanding of *qi* that runs counter to students' translations. This statement underscores the ways in which the students are now participants in the translation of Chinese medicine. When they use terms like "energy," for example, they participate in the perpetuation of a certain idea of *qi*, one that is inaccurate according to experts, and potentially concealing. Carter is further teaching a strategy of participation wherein the students are challenged to know what multiple English-language speaking experts have to say:

> Carter: We can think of *qi* as sort of *subtle* materials, or *mobile in*fluences. Ah, maybe somewhere between matter (.) and non-matter. Um (4.7) Unschuld (.), the historian, commonly translates *qi* to be—If he's gonna bother translating it, he talks about it in terms of=as *in*fluences, right? Vital influences on the body (0.8)—not, not influence? But influen*ces*, right, plural.

Here, Carter explains *qi* by using multiple expert sources, including both Kaptchuk (without citation)[1] and Unschuld, to describe the phenomenon in English, as well as to talk about what it means to translate the term. These scholars, we have observed in the previous two chapters, draw upon vastly different ideologies of translation themselves, but here they are paired together for the purpose of classroom translation. This offers an example of the way in which everyday translation emerges in an ongoing conversation involving multiple texts and multiple participants. By focusing on the choice made by these scholars, it also effectively initiates students' into the practice of translation as replete with strategic choices and personal decisions about which terms to use. Carter also instructs them in a strategy of translation that privileges a comprehensive knowledge of expert sources, at once establishing his own grounds of authority by citing such sources and challenging students, as novice participants, to do the same.

Carter goes on to cite other expert authors, drawing upon their translations both to teach about *qi* and to teach about the complexities of translation. Showing these other options for translating *qi* demonstrates the difficulty of translating in Chinese medicine, as well as it highlights the strategy of doing so with a strong foundation in diverse sources. He finishes by again emphasizing this difficulty:

> Carter: So we start to see (0.8) it's difficult to translate. There's different aspects of it, ok? And because of that, we find, it's generally not=people don't bother. Well, it's *qi*. Let's just call it *qi*. And that way it has all these multiple layered meanings to it.

People do not bother to translate *qi*, Carter explains, because there are so many aspects to the term. Most authors therefore use the borrowed term. This way, Carter explains, the term retains all of its multiple meanings. With this final statement, students are socialized into the use of borrowed terms and the imagined impossibility of translation.

In this segment, students are introduced to the contingency of translation in Chinese medicine, including the notion that it is acceptable for all the authorities to talk about it differently. Carter participates in this contingency by offering different explanations, drawing upon available texts and scholarly authorities, and claiming none of them as the only right one. This strategy is Carter's conscious engagement in teaching translation. With this strategy, he establishes his own authority, as a Caucasian male who does not speak Chinese, to translate for students, using reported speech to establish evidence that his claims are "already co-constructed" (Hill and Irvine 1993: 7), as well as possibly to mitigate his own accountability in a field of uncertainty (Pomerantz 1984). Because he intimately knows all of these authoritative sources who *do* speak Chinese well, he is able to make claims about how to interact with the available evidence. This strategy is related to Carter's understanding of his role as teacher. "My job," he says in the first class, "is to just tell you what's out there, make sure that you know all the different [translations]." Carter's own teaching philosophy thus incorporates an articulated perspective on translation and how best to teach students how to engage with the complexity of multiple English-language translations. This perspective offers students a certain kind of agency in relation to translation, empowering them with the choice and awareness of multiple English-language expert opinions as well as the sense that, in choosing from amongst these opinions, they are themselves participating in the translation of Chinese medicine into spoken English. This strategy for both describing and ultimately performing translation emerges in a classroom interaction that involves Carter, the students, as well as the authors that Carter cites as evidence. All of these parties, each with their own strategies for translation and claims to legitimacy, participate in a dialogic encounter wherein the source term, *qi*, is translated into English through a discussion of multiple translations and explanations.

More Talk about Qi

The next two examples demonstrates how, in living translation, interactions about translation, and the concurrent ongoing performance of translation, extend beyond the classroom. Taken from interviews, these examples show two students, Julia and Oren, engaging in the dialogue about translating *qi*. It is apparent that their articulations are based in a core resistance to the translation strategies they are taught in class. Not only do their perspectives reveal the ongoing nature of interactions concerning translation, they show how students learn very early on in their education to participate in the translation of Chinese medicine, actively finding diverse evidence for their own socially and morally grounded ways of authoritatively understanding and interpreting Chinese language.

The first interview segment is taken from a conversation with Julia, quoted in part in chapter 1 and revisited extensively in chapter 2, where her views on the lack of necessity for the translation of *qi* into any specific English term are viewed in light of the moral frameworks and ideologies of language informing her views on translation. Here, I offer longer excerpts from the interview to demonstrate that her perspective on the translation of this term is one that is formed in interaction with Carter. Referring to the segment quoted in the first example, Julia discusses the "conversation" that they were having about how to translate *qi* in her class:

> Like, you know, just in the last class, we were having this conversation about *qi*, about how there's really like no tran—there's no, you know—Carter was going on and on and on ((laughing)) about like how there's no um, there's no direct translation for *qi*.

Here, Julia's designation of the classroom interaction as a "conversation" is interesting in that, although it was indeed interactive, it only involved one or two comments from the students. The rest was Carter lecturing, or as Julia puts it, "going on and on." The fact that Julia characterizes it as a conversation, however, highlights the fact that even in situations where the teacher is primarily lecturing to students, students are always responding, whether they speak or not. In the interview, Julia describes her response to Carter's lecture:

> And he gave us this *huge* list of like all the trans—Possible trans—you know, all the translations from different sources—And all this *stuff* about how—but then ultimately, you know, twenty minutes later what we of course came to is that, you know, *qi* is *qi.* And you can't translate it because it is its own thing. It's its own entity. Whatever. And it's like *duh,* you know, of *course, NEXT SLIDE,* you know? ((laughing))

Exaggerating a bit with the "twenty minutes" comment, Julia characterizes Carter's citation of multiple experts as unnecessary with the statement that "of course … *qi* is *qi.*" Here, it is interesting to note the "of course," as if it were obvious to her that *qi* is none other than, simply, *qi.* She emphasizes this again by saying "like duh, you know, of *course, NEXT SLIDE,* you know?" using sarcasm and "you know?" (twice) to make it clear that the lack of a direct translation for *qi* was not news to her. This causes her to question the need for even the short explanation that Carter offered. With her exaggerations, she is also mocking his teaching and his translation strategy, contesting the need to examine multiple sources and translations to explain *qi* and simultaneously questioning his authority. From here she gets into describing her own ideas about translation strategies:

> What the hell, like, I mean, you know, I feel that way about a *ton* of these words. Like, you know, who cares? Like call it *LAMP* if you want to. You know what I mean? Like, it's an *idea.* It's an *idea,* it's a—it's a *thing,* you know, it's an id—it's its own kind of *idea.* So we don't need to—we can call it anything we want.

Julia, at least at this stage in her education, clearly has the feeling that language, as far as specific terms go, is arbitrary. In her view, it is the idea that is primary, a perspective that leads to her loose translation strategy that, as we see below, depends on changing explanations and multiple uses of the word "like," rather than precise terms. Julia's evidence for this strategy of "not translating" is her moral experience both of *qi* and of language in the world:

> It's like *God,* you know what I mean? Like how many wars and like everything over the *word God,* and like, is it this kind of—Is it like when you say God, though, ((in foreign accent)) What do you mean? Is it like *exactly* the type of God that I am? ((laughing)) It's like, you know (.) and now we're coming to more understanding of the world. That like—and you know, like, even in conversation people say God, or nature, or whatever—you know, people are starting to be more sensitive to that reality that people are so hung up on the *word.*

Here, Julia compares *qi* to "the *word God,*" which according to her is the root of much of the world's problems. She mocks a foreign accent while she quotes an unspecified other, and notably links war to misunderstandings based in language rather than true meaning. True meaning, she suggests, is not linked to language, and "we're coming to more understanding of the world" where complex ideas like God or nature are supposedly equivalent. She separates herself from "people" who are "so hung up on the *word,*" again distinguishing herself from the Other/foreigner and aligning herself with the stance that language is arbitrary. For Julia, this strongly articulated view of translation wherein "the word" is somehow separate from the meaning is an extremely moral position linked to an evolutionary assessment of the increasing recognition of the difference between reality, or ideas, and language. Because she aligns herself with the stance that language does not matter as much as meaning, she gets annoyed and frustrated when language is brought up in class:

> It's just I don't like having those conversations in class. It annoys me, it frustrates me, I think it's like we are, like, so *off* the mark? When we're talking about that? You know? We're *so* like not talking about the point, here? When we're trying to figure out like what the, like, what *qi*—like what that *exact* sound would translate to in English is like. It feels to me like it's like an apples and oranges kind of conversation, you know? And I wish that we weren't even encouraged to pursue that? You know, route. I don't see any reason to try and *force* that into a word that we already have in English. Doesn't seem necessary. It is *qi*. Learn it. It's the *new medicine,* you know, here it is.

Based on her earlier statements, the "mark," as she calls it, would be centered more around the idea of *qi* rather than the translation for *qi*, and she clearly states this when she explains that finding the "exact sound" in English feels like "an apples and oranges kind of conversation." Again, she is criticizing a teaching method that incorporates discussion of language, when the "new medicine" is based in a moral-evolutionary position that transcends language. In this sense, she argues that the ideal role for her (and others) in the dialogue about translation is to refrain from debate. On the surface, then, it may appear that she is refusing to engage in the discussion. However, the very articulation of this strong opinion on translation is itself a form of participation in the overall dialogue *about* translation. It is also apparent that, in taking this extreme stance, Julia, a massage therapist, is also herself translating:

> When people—like what is this heat going through my body? I mean I always tell like people, like clients and stuff when they're like what is that? And I'm like, it's *qi* ° They're like what's *qi*? And I'll be like, aw, *qi*'s kind of like your universal life force energy—It's all in the *world,* it's coming *in you,* it's going *out of you.* It's like, you know, it's makin' things happen, it *is* those things that are happening, like, and

> it is that *heat* that you are feeling in you ankle right now—And people are like *OH*. And it's like it—because it is a thing in the world? It's like, people aren't like well what is it in English? I mean no one has *ever* asked me that, none of my clients, like, regardless of their orientation.

When her massage clients ask her about their embodied experience, she explains it as "it's *qi*" with a rising intonation. The rising intonation underscores her certainty that the sensations felt by her clients are, plainly, *qi*. In one sense, by using the term *qi*, she is refusing to translate. She does, however, go on to explain *qi* to her clients using more detailed language: "it's kind of like your universal life force energy." Here, she is not only providing an English gloss in an epistemically downgraded way ("kind of like your"), but it is clear that she is also "doing" translation, simultaneously positioning herself in a moral world where precise language does not matter. She continues with this loose definition by saying "it's all in the world, it's coming in you, it's going out of you, it's like you know, it's makin' things happen, it is those things that are happening," generating her own intralingual circumlocution to represent the foreign term. Her words here indicate that *qi* might not have a very precise definition, but that she understands the concept perfectly well, and like other U.S. students who despite claiming that *qi* can only be understood vis-à-vis embodied experience are still able to talk about it (Ho 2004), has no problem explaining it in English. She finishes this explanation by saying that "it is that *heat* that you are feeling in your ankle right now." This particular part of her explanation shows that Julia uses embodied evidence to understand and explain *qi*, positioning herself as an expert with no need to pay attention to the sources Carter cites in class. In so doing, she participates in an ongoing interaction that enacts the translation of the term *qi* and is very much mediated by Julia's moral and ideological commitments.

In this example, we see that Julia, even in her first quarter, has begun to think seriously about translation in relation to the terms she is learning in class. Her response also indicates the extent to which she understands herself as an agent of translation, as well as a participant in the dialogue about translation in Chinese medicine. Indeed, she *is* a participant in the sense that she translates Chinese terms for massage clients and does so based on a highly articulated translation strategy. The fact that this strategy differs significantly from the one she is taught in class shows that, regardless of what specific words are chosen or agreed upon, in living translation there is often resistance and variation in explanation and understanding as participants use translation to position themselves as authorities. These variables emerge clearly when we look closely at the way translation unfolds in interactive spaces, such as those created between Julia and her massage clients or between Julia and her teachers. Even as a novice, then, Julia is a participant in the conversation by which *qi* is translated into the United States. This clearly raises concerns about the one-sided nature of the conversation. Julia, in refusing to consider how experts have translated this key term, here shows us that she has perhaps not yet begun really to learn how to listen with much discernment to the many voices telling her how to translate or how not to translate Chinese medical terms, as the case may be. As we shall see, however, this changes over the course of her education.

In the following excerpt, parts of which have also appeared in previous chapters, Oren, in his third quarter, similarly reflects upon the translation of *qi*, but with a much different attitude and a much different translation:

> I would translate it as vitality. And then within that translation make all the necessary subcategories of it—subtranslations.

In this excerpt, Oren uses the words "I would" when discussing his perspective on the translation of *qi*. These words suggest that he does not necessarily actually make this translational choice *yet,* but if Oren were in the position of translator (and indeed, once he is in that position with patients), he would and he will make that choice. In a sense, then, Oren is describing how he would do translation, but it is also clear that in making the above statement, Oren *is* participating in translation by choosing "vitality," an uncommon and relatively unique gloss, to translate *qi*. The choice to translate the term using this quick and easy, though uncommon, English word demonstrates the position that translation can be a simple and straightforward process. Oren thus advocates a translation strategy that embraces such simple glosses. He continues with this perspective by saying that he would then "make all the necessary subcategories of it—subtranslations," suggesting that further explication of the term in English would be equally clear-cut and uncomplicated. This translation strategy is based in a strongly affective stance:

> But I don't like that it's still *qi* in English. I think it should be vitality. I think *yin* and *yang* should have their own English words.

In this part of the example, Oren shows that his translation strategy is tied to personal preferences, what he likes and does not like. The "still" here further indexes a temporality that suggests the term *qi* is out-of-date, that perhaps it lingers from an earlier, less refined time. This is the first indication in this excerpt that Oren's stance on translation is based in a complex series of judgments, for example that Chinese words such as *qi, yin,* and *yang* "should" have English equivalents. When I question this stance, Oren links language to cultural authority:

> I don't think we should be running around using *pinyin*. Because that gives the Chinese an authority. This is the—English is the language that I'll be using in this

culture, and if there are Chinese words thrown in here and there for the most important concepts? Then Chinese people will always have the authority.

This portion of the excerpt was cited above, in relation to the ideology of language as cultural capital. What is relevant here is that, already for Oren in his third quarter, translation is a site at which one can assert one's authority through language. This affective, moral stance clearly affects the ways in which he undertakes the project of translation, urging him to seek straightforward English glosses like "vitality" to translate Chinese terms. This excerpt reveals Oren's sense of participation in the conversation about translation and shows him using an affective, moral authority as the basis to understand and translate *qi*. He is an agent in this discussion, with the ability to make choices that differ from those made by prominent authorities, including teachers and authors. Such choices emerge out of and give rise to definite strategies that are not only heavily mediated by historical, institutional, and moral forces, but also impact the way Chinese medicine is translated in Oren's (future) practice.

These two segments demonstrate the ways in which textual translations and classroom interactions can cause students to think more deeply about translation. In addition to sparking an awareness of the contingency of the information in their texts, such interactions awaken the students' awareness that to access a truth that makes sense to them and that they can legitimately present to patients and colleagues, they must participate in the discussion themselves. As Treavor says once he becomes an intern in the community clinic, "You cannot NOT translate." This statement underscores the importance of learning and doing translation as a skill equally as important as learning to feel patients' pulses and prescribing formulas. The segments shown here thus demonstrate the ways in which interactions in the classroom are one point along an ongoing continuum of living translation as it occurs in an American school of Chinese medicine. Along this continuum, students make critical decisions about who they listen to, when, and how they listen. These choices directly affect the ways in which they participate in the conversation and the ways in which they thus enact translation.

Translation in Interaction II: Rheum for Interpretation

In the next set of examples, many of the same students discussed in the first part of this chapter are in a third-quarter class on organ theory in Chinese medicine. In this instance, Dr. Liu, a Mainland Chinese doctor of Chinese medicine, responds to questions his students have regarding the English term "rheum," a translation for the term 饮 *yin,* phonetically the same as 阴 *yin* of the well-known *yin-yang,* however the meaning and orthography of the characters differ considerably. Briefly, rheum is defined as pathological fluid in the body, thinner than "phlegm" (痰 *tan*) and manifesting in multiple ways depending on the affected organ (Wiseman and Feng 1998: 440). Outside the term "rheumatoid arthritis," the term is not commonly used in colloquial English, most likely the reason why it was chosen by Wiseman and Feng as a translation for *yin*. Wiseman and Feng's translation philosophy, discussed extensively in the previous two chapters, encourages students of Chinese medicine to learn unfamiliar terms to use as technical terms in their practice. The aim of this strategy is to prevent readers from too easily associating the meanings of familiar words with the meanings of these specialized terms. Rheum is one such specialized term and therefore only appears in select texts. In the following sets of excerpts, I show the many ways in which this term emerges from the texts and into conversation in multiple contexts where teachers and students participate in an ongoing set of interactions that, together with the texts, enact the translation of this term.

The Meaning of Rheum

In the first set of excerpts, the first-year students are in their third-quarter class on organ theory in Chinese medicine. Dr. Liu, their Chinese instructor, responds to questions posed by his students, who have just been introduced to the term "rheum" in their teacher-constructed notebook. This notebook, in contrast to texts, is an unofficial supplement to the required texts. As such, the language included in this notebook (as in others provided by different teachers) differs quite considerably from official texts. Because rheum is not in any of their other texts, the students struggle to figure out exactly what this word means in the context of their current knowledge. About thirty-five minutes into class, Tanya, one of the students, questions Dr. Liu about this term:

Tanya:	Doctor? (0.4)
Dr. Liu:	Yes
Tanya:	What is rheum? R-H-E-U-M? (1.2)
	((Oren is whispering in background))
Dr. Liu:	R-H-E-U-N-E-U-M, yeah.
Tanya:	R-H-E-U-M.
Dr. Liu:	Rheum.
Tanya:	I've never seen that before.

From the beginning of this interaction, Tanya topicalizes rheum. She continues her questioning of the term by spelling it out for the teacher, indexing her lack of familiarity with the term and perhaps distinguishing it from the more common "room." She makes this lack of familiarity explicit by saying that she has never seen it before. Her tone here suggests that it might be a complaint or at the very least that her lack of familiarity demands an explanation from the teacher. This initiates a sequence in which multiple parties, including Dr. Liu as well as two other students, Oren and Julia, become involved in a discussion about translation:

Dr. Liu: Sure. I check the (2.0.)
Oren: ((whispering)) It's mucus
Dr. Liu: Chinese medicine dictionary, that's in our library
Tanya: Uh-huh
Dr. Liu: E:h—actually translated it=because that word in Chinese called *yin*. (0.6)
((Julia removes her Chinese dictionary from her bag and opens it))

Here, Dr. Liu indicates that for him, as well as for Tanya, the concept of *yin* presents a translation problem. Instead of offering Tanya an explanation of the *meaning* of the term, however, Dr. Liu offers an explanation of his difficulties in finding an appropriate translation, difficulties that led him to the dictionary in the school library, itself only one of many dictionaries translating Chinese medicine into English. The choice to explain it this way could indicate that Dr. Liu thinks Tanya understands the English word but is just searching for what it means in Chinese. He therefore starts peeling back the translation and uses the Chinese to clarify, appealing to the dictionary as evidence for the validity of his translation. He promptly interrupts his own explanation, however, by referencing the Chinese word *yin* as the ultimate evidence. This code-switch to Chinese works to position Dr. Liu as an authority who can access the Chinese and who can thereby speak about what should constitute the evidence for translational (as well as clinical) decisions. It also begins to signal one of the major ideologies of language operating behind Dr. Liu's teaching strategy, namely, the ideology of language as inherently indexical of a semantic network that provides access to the classics or at least to some Chinese texts.

The use of Chinese creates further confusion, however, as the students for the most part do not read or write Chinese and are clearly struggling to understand the meaning of rheum in English rather than Chinese. This is apparent in Oren's gloss, when he loudly whispers, "It's mucus" to his neighboring classmates. This statement demonstrates Oren's resistance to the more detailed explanation being concurrently offered by the teacher, indexing his preference for a quick translational gloss that disregards the complex implications of translation and displaces cultural authority. Similarly, when Julia gets out her pocket-size Chinese dictionary and attempts to figure it out for herself, this action indicates a certain lack of clarity or understanding based on the teacher's explanation, as well as indicating her growing desire, developed over the course of two quarters, to learn as much Chinese as she can. In both of these cases, the students are actively participating in the translation of *yin* for themselves as well as for those around them, especially observable later in the class when several students lean over Julia's dictionary to see what she has found. Meanwhile, Dr. Liu continues his translation endeavor by explaining the term in relation to a series of neighboring Chinese medical concepts, including 痰 *tan* (phlegm) and 水肿 *shui zhong* (edema), and differentiating it from these conditions by saying that it lies somewhere "between" the two. This differentiation demonstrates his ideology of language, wherein specific words are mere indexes of a whole network of concepts that link the terms together, especially through classical texts. This ideology contrasts significantly with both Oren's and Julia's ideologies of language, and more confusion ensues as Dr. Liu invokes the authority of the standard textbooks in China, presumably to back up the importance of his claim that the students know the concept of *yin*/rheum:

> Dr. Liu: Ah, the rheum (.) in the fundamental book=internal medicine book, no translation Ah, no translation ((smiling)) Also in Chinese medicine—the standard textbook (0.2) it's a major part also ((laughs briefly)) So I don't know why they miss that.

Here, Dr. Liu complains about the English texts and the fact that they do not include a translation for *yin*. He passes judgment on this lack of translation, complaining that in the standard Chinese books "it's a major part also." This statement is followed by a laugh that underscores the egregiousness of the offense that English language authors, deictically referenced as "they," commit when they neglect to include the term in their books. Later in the class, Dr. Liu's use of the Chinese texts as sufficient evidence for the necessity of this concept is resisted by several students, who continue to be suspicious of a concept that does not appear in their main textbooks. One of these students, Todd, complains that since "none of my other classes have mentioned this," he does not understand how to approach the conditions with herbs. He proceeds then to press Dr. Liu to name an English textbook that discusses this term:

> Todd: And which book? Is there, is there a book, ah?
> Dr. Liu: Ah, in Chinese book.
> Todd: Only Chinese book.
> Dr. Liu: Anything—every textbook, they have this part. Only in English book, they don't have it.

Although it is not immediately readable from the transcript, Todd's tone here is irreverent. For example, Todd mocks the Dr. Liu's response by using the singular "book" instead of books. His intonation here suggests a complaint that he does not have access to the Chinese books and further indicates his expectation that the information should be translated into English for him to digest and use in practice. Dr. Liu defends his position here, and in so doing manages to accomplish several things. Firstly, he defends his position of authority in the classroom based on his knowledge of Chinese texts. Secondly, he defends himself to Todd. Thirdly, he defends the authority of the Chinese texts as opposed to the English texts and overtly criticizes the English texts for failing to include crucial information.

In a further act of resistance, Oren here cuts in, asking, "Is it a subcategory of dampness?" With this question, Oren seeks to place rheum in a known taxonomy of the body. Dr. Liu answers negatively, insisting that *yin* is not "sub" to anything:

> Dr. Liu: That's very independent syndrome (.) For example, you have Bell's Palsy syndrome (.) that fall into a neurological disease in Western medicine? But Bell's Palsy also very *special* syndrome (1.2) They just syndrome—special—so rheum is like that (.) Very special.

Here, Dr. Liu refuses to accept Oren's recategorization of the term, using the taxonomy of biomedicine to make his point. Rheum, he explains, is like Bell's Palsy, an independent syndrome that deserves its own translation. Here, the frustration in the class escalates, however, as the students begin to grow even more restless and confused. In conversation with Oren later, I was informed that part of the difficulty stemmed from the fact that he, along with several of his classmates seated near him, thought that Dr. Liu had not understood his question and that perhaps rheum was a subcategory of dampness after all.

Amidst all the confusion, however, Tanya requests that Dr. Liu write the character for *yin* on the board for them. This proves an interesting discussion in light of the fact that the students, for the most part, do not write or read Chinese. In one sense, it reveals that many of the students are eager to learn the Chinese names for things and do honestly consider Chinese language to be the ultimate source of knowledge in Chinese medicine. However, it also demonstrates that many of them are challenged by Dr. Liu's interpretive strategies and are trying to map a better translation on their own. For a good twenty minutes, then, the class is embedded in an extensive discussion of the character for *yin* as well as several other surrounding characters that Dr. Liu insists are crucial to understand how to translate the term properly. At this point, the term "rheum" is all but abandoned.

This example offers several insights into the dynamics of translation in the school context. First, it shows how Dr. Liu draws upon divergent ideologies of language in translation as well as clinically important notions of meaning and evidence to interactively establish his authority in the social field of U.S. Chinese medicine. Because the ultimate authoritative sources are in Chinese and not otherwise available to the students, who cannot read them, this example shows Dr. Liu positioning himself as a gatekeeper to the Chinese, an authority whose English is often challengeable, but whose Chinese is not. Second, the interaction demonstrates that Dr. Liu understands and seeks to teach clinical decision-making through translation. Here, the evidence that he offers as providing the ground for diagnosis, is, again, the Chinese textual canon. This not only reinforces his authority but provides him also with a platform for his introduction to the notion of what language is and should be in Chinese medicine: an entry point into a systematic understanding of the body and world.

Dr. Liu is not the only actor here, however. The interaction also offers students an opportunity to participate in translation, as they resist and contest Dr. Liu's strategies for handling the translation of *yin* at the same time as they resist his authority and socialize him into their own ideologies of language. Thus, from the beginning of this sequence, it is clear that disparate ideologies of translation, different *demands* of translation, can instigate struggle in the classroom. This "clash of ideologies" continues throughout the remainder of the class, as Oren, Tanya, and other students continue to wrestle with the term, attempting to classify it in terms of the knowledge included in their primary, English-language texts. In the end, *yin* is translated vis-à-vis multiple explanations of the character, multiple explanations of neighboring concepts, and multiple suggestions of English equivalents, none of which prove to be completely satisfying. Taken as a whole, this sequence aptly demonstrates the process of living translation as enacted through interaction, as an unfolding process with implications far beyond "language" as narrowly conceived.

Rheum for Play

The next set of examples demonstrates a further evidential strategy for teaching and performing translation and suggests a possible reason for the students' struggle with Dr. Liu's insistence on the translation "rheum," although this insight is not confirmed. Like the first two examples, it occurs interactively in a classroom moment that involves students, teachers, and authors as coparticipants. In this case, Barbara—the teacher cited in the opening quote for this chapter and mentioned repeatedly in other chapters—uses the translated terms "loins" and "rheum" as platforms for establishing her authority to translate based on an authentic cultural and aesthetic appeal. The segment takes place in the students' second quarter, three or four months prior to the example above. Most of the same students are in the class—Julia, Oren, Todd, and others. It begins with Barbara's use of a certain characteristic playfulness to approach the term *loins,* a term used in the teacher-provided text to talk about the location where the students might feel cold on their patients' bodies:

Barbara: Alright, next place we'll look for cold is, um—(0.6) ((turns to whiteboard and begins to write)) ((turning her head back)) like a gothic romance novel (1.2) ((in deeper voice)) her *loins* were *cold.* (1.6) ((students laugh))

In contrast to the previous example, this excerpt occurs in what Goffman (1974) might call a "play frame" as Barbara dramatically classifies the term *loins* as reminiscent of an entirely different genre of text than they are studying in class, namely a "gothic romance novel." This drama is evident with the tossing of her head back and the sultry voice she affects to communicate an example of "loins" as used in a trashy novel. This drama instantly engages the students in a shared moment where certain American cultural understandings are made explicit. In its linking of the language used in their textbooks with the language used in novels, it also draws them in to a discussion of translation:

Barbara: The Chinese are still translating, or whoever's translating for them are still translating things, ah, like, um, ((students laugh)) loins and lumbago, and ((waving arms upward)) (1.2) rheum, and (.) different kinds of (.) things that you really only see either in a meat market or in a gothic (.) romance (.) novel ((students laugh)) like a harlequin romance.

In this part of the segment, Barbara continues to involve the students by maintaining a playful dramatic stance that hinges upon their participation as audience members who "get" her references. In so doing, she teaches translation as something dependent upon the audience and their popular cultural knowledge, revealing translation choices as "funny" and antiquated when they evoke certain cultural images like meat markets or harlequin novels. This perspective simultaneously invokes the notion that translators who "still" use these common terms to translate are stuck in the (vulgar?) past, where language about the human body was embedded in discourses of sex and romance. This not only echoes an ideology of language that locates truth in nature as separated from language, but also foreshadows the positioning that Barbara will take as the arbiter of knowledge that must be extracted from these sticky translations.

This strategy is not arbitrary. With it, Barbara positions herself as an authority capable of interpreting the silly translation choices of "the Chinese ... or whoever's translating for them" to the students. This is especially interesting, considering the source of the term (loins) that sparks this discussion is her own teacher-provided text, which is based on a translation, likely for the term 腰 *yao* (waist or small of back), found in a text translated by a British scholar working for English and American audiences (Maciocia 2005). Furthermore, the use of "rheum" as a further example for the (crazy? old-fashioned?) Chinese translations is surprising considering Barbara's familiarity with rheum as the Wiseman-Feng translation for *yin*, a fact she references in a later class. Despite this, the accuracy of the statement matters less than the work it is doing in the moment to position Barbara in relation to the source of Chinese medicine. So whereas Dr. Liu establishes his authority based on his access to Chinese language and texts, Barbara establishes her authority based on a cultural knowledge of the students, using things like gothic romance novels and meat markets to translate concepts for them. In so doing, Barbara also offers the students a way to relate to unfamiliar English terms by showing them that they are not necessarily technical terms but are instead drawn from specific and outdated genres of writing. In addition to positioning Barbara as expert interpreter, this not only functions to draw the students into a world of "us" and "them," but further reinforces the notion that the ultimate basis for their diagnostic activities should be founded not on unreliable translations, but on the universal and unchanging human body. Ironically, Barbara then performs this universality by pointing to her own buttocks and using a culturally specific term (roast) to identify what the terms under discussion "actually" mean:

> Barbara: So when they talk about loins (.) if we go back to the meat market (.) ((one student snickers)) we're actually talking about that area ((pointing to her hip/buttocks)) that makes a good roast, (0.6) right?

Here, Barbara uses deictic referencing to demonstrate the act of translation, positioning "the Chinese or whoever" as the talkers and "us" (herself and her students) as the interpreters. In other words, *they* talk about things, but *we* must participate, using our experience to interpret their talk. This statement initiates students into a dialogic relationship with translators where their voices must be heard against the backdrop of students' cultural experience. Her use of the word "actually," when she says that "we're actually talking about," utilizes this ideology to contrastively accomplish the work of translation intersemiotically vis-à-vis her own embodied stance and the cultural awareness of what parts of the body make a good roast. It further indexes an ideology of language that locates language, especially the language of Chinese translators, somewhere far apart from the lived reality of the body.

This set of excerpts offers another illustration of the ways in which translation in the context of American schools is accomplished in interactive moments that involve teachers, students, and authors in dialogic encounters where translation talk becomes a site for participants to establish their authority, to socialize students into various ways of finding and interpreting evidence, and to introduce and articulate various ideologies of language that will impact the way they make choices in practice. As the last example shows, such encounters are not always seamless. Conflict arises as translation strategies are measured against one another and found deficient for various reasons. In this case, it is Barbara who takes issue with "the Chinese or whoever is translating for them," arguing that their persistent use of outdated terms more appropriate to harlequin romance novels than to Chinese medicine complicates the translation process and makes it difficult to understand the texts. From this vantage point, the material requires a further level of intralingual translation or explanation, as well as intersemiotic translation in the form of embodied display, to make it meaningful for users, and Barbara steps comfortably into that role As an example of living translation, the excerpts here reveal the social *work* that is done with talk about translation and suggest the ways in which translation talk is used to direct students' clinical practice of diagnosis, in this case guiding them away from the terminology and toward the human body as the source of relevant information about illness.

Rheum for Reflection

Barbara's casual dismissal of terms like loins and rheum perhaps contributes to the students difficulty in appreciating Dr. Liu's later insistence on the importance of rheum as a key concept in Chinese medicine. Interestingly, however, the conflict in Dr. Liu's classroom generates a great deal of reflectiveness in many of the participants. Follow-up interviews offer a great deal of insight into how deeply such moments of confusion, perhaps even more than moments of clarity, influence the students' ideas about translation and encourage them to develop a strong discursive consciousness about translation. Treavor, who was home sick from Dr. Liu's class the day of the rheum discussion, hears about the conflict from Julia and Sarah and comments to me about it in an interview. He says that this "thing" that they are studying, this thing "that we call medicine," is also to a certain extent "history":

> History isn't a matter of what the truth is. History is a matter of what people in power *decide* other people should know ... So in the process of taking this medicine from the East and bringing it to the West, there are all kinds of decisions that get made along the way that have nothing to do with the medicine.

This comment reveals the ways in which interactions like those described above cause students to think more deeply about the language they are learning and can spark an awareness of the contingency of the information in their texts. In this case, translation talk works to interrupt the common ideology of language as factual, introducing students to a world in which language is fundamentally social and historical. For Treavor, it provides an opportunity to strengthen his deeply felt ideology of learning that places his own experience at the center of interpretive truth. "Ultimately," he says in another interview, "because I'm the one who's going to be in charge of my own practice, I just need to learn from—all [of the different translations out there]." For other students, however, the instability that emerges from such conflicts inspires resistance and confusion. Tricia, the French student quoted in chapter 2 as talking about her inability to intuitively grasp Chinese concepts, actually drops out once she realizes that there is no way to fit Chinese medical terms into the neat little "drawers" that she had become accustomed to in her undergrad pre-med training. And Oren, who argues for a simple translation for *qi* in the first set of examples as well as for a straightforward gloss for *yin* ("mucus") in the second, never ends up succeeding in his quest for the one-to-one translation. In a later interview, he complains that Dr. Liu's English was probably not good enough to understand his superior translation. Sarah, on the other hand, who was present for both segments, says about the conflict that "I think it's just really opening my eyes to the limitations of translation." Conflicts like the one in Dr. Liu's class remind her that learning Chinese medicine is "like being a baby and learning a new language, where you really just have to be open to the language and not try to parallel it to what we already know." Unlike Oren, Sarah here demonstrates an ideology of translation that refuses to accept simple correspondences and strives to achieve a deep, childlike listening. In this sense, language becomes for Sarah an access point to a parallel world and not at all a referentially transparent index of either a universally experienced reality or body-self.

The effects of such conflicts do not necessarily ever end. In fact, in even further interviews down the line, Julia says two years later, when she is an intern, that she finally understands what rheum is based on her experiences in the clinic. "I mean I do get now what it is," she says. "But I had to see it to, to believe it, to know." She goes on to describe her experience of rheum, saying that it is a "snotty but not snot, like phlegmy but not phlegm-dampy but not exactly damp, like sort of *thing* that is in somebody." She reiterates that she must see it to truly get it, however, and only then can she communicate about it with her teachers and supervisors, who also know what it is through experience. She refers back to the day in Dr. Liu's class cited above as "the whole hilarious outburst about [rheum]":

> When we first heard the word that was just of no sense-making, and it could not be explained to us exactly what this substance *was*. So we have a very comfortable, even intimate and close, like you know, association with the word rheum. Because it really was this whole thing for us to get over the learning of it.

Here, Julia references the intimate relationship that she has with language in Chinese medicine, in particular the word "rheum," which was the source of so much discussion about translation back in her first year. As I demonstrate in the next chapter, this type of intimacy is the foundation for an embodied understanding of language in the living translation of Chinese medicine. It also highlights how experience with the terminology in practice changes Julia's overall experience of language and meaning in Chinese medicine:

> It is fun to have such a relationship with it. I would say of all the terms we've used, that's the one that it's like been the most [fun] for us to watch our own develop-

> ment with it? Because it like almost has like a—it feels like, like every time we use the word it's like oh my God, I can't believe it, I'm gonna—I'm givin' over, I'm usin' the crazy word. Because like it's a real thing, and so to like really acknowledge that? You know … is sort of a, it's sort of amazing. When we were like "this word doesn't even exist."

Here, we hear Julia experiencing a rereading of a term that, prior to her experience in the clinic "seeing" rheum, did not even exist for her. In this sense, the translation provided by Dr. Liu vis-à-vis the Wiseman-Feng dictionary ends up attaining legitimacy in Julia's repertoire, despite being dismissed by her other teacher, Barbara, as well as her classmates. Two years down the line, Julia expresses an "epideictic clarity" (Crapanzano 2011) regarding rheum that demonstrates the ways in which interactions about translation in Chinese medicine are ongoing endeavors that extend directly into the moralized realm of experience and penetrate also the ways in which the medicine is practiced. While this experience does not necessarily change her basic ideology of language as an arbitrary signifier of a higher truth, it certainly expands upon it and can be said to move it at least a little more toward the language-as-network approach that Dr. Liu tries to teach ("snotty but not snot, phlegmy but not phlegm-dampy but not exactly damp"). In many ways, it also legitimates Dr. Liu's authority many years after the fact and introduces the reality of rheum into Julia's clinical practice. In this sense, Julia's process of "learning how to listen" in living translation emerges through an interaction that spans several years and that deeply involves her own clinical experience as well as conversations with experts and the study of Chinese language.

Discussion and Conclusion

In this chapter, I have shown several classroom interactions about translation and talk in which teachers use different evidentiality strategies, ranging from the direct quoting of sources to the use of personal and cultural experience as evidence for and against certain translations. I have shown also the ways in which translation talk unfolds over time as a social process with potential implications for clinical practice. Together, these data suggest that translation in U.S. Chinese medical education advances as a conversation in constant motion, a hermeneutic endeavor in which the translation and explanation of foreign terms is always interactively mediated by the use of different kinds of evidence to epistemically position participants with regard to a set of imagined originals, the different moral demands of participants, as well as the multiple ideologies of language and translation circulating in this complex field. Within these ongoing conversations, multiple texts and other cultural, experiential, and linguistic sources are drawn upon to talk about and accomplish translation in an interactive setting involving multiple parties with divergent moral and linguistic strategies for both listening and translating. This lends a quality of "multi-voicedness" to such interactions, wherein multiple participants are discursively interpreting multiple sources, and each utterance about translated material reflects the intention of the speaker as well as the "refracted intention" of the translator, the original author, and all of the divergent interpretations that the speaker has been exposed to (Bakhtin 1981: 324). In addition to this, the interactions that lead ultimately to the translation of Chinese medical terms are always ongoing, as participants leave the classroom to translate and retranslate in various contexts. The result is, in the words of Octavio Paz, "a symphony in which improvisation is inseparable from translation and creation is indistinguishable from imitation" (1992 [1971]: 160–161). In living translation, Chinese medicine is translated via this "symphony" of multiple, complex strategies in interaction with one another. In the context of American Chinese medical education, *qi* becomes alternately "energy," "vitality," "breaths," "life force," or "that heat in your ankle," among other things. *Yin* becomes "rheum," "mucus," "something between phlegm and edema," and "snot but not snot, phlegmy but not phlegm-dampy," and the never-mentioned Chinese word for loins become "that part of your body that makes a good roast."

In considering these multiple voices, it is important to keep in mind the complex social politics of translation in Chinese medicine, including the ongoing tensions between ideologies of incommensurability and source-based translation, clashes between institutionally motivated translations and independently constructed interpretations meant to challenge existing institutions. From this perspective, one could argue that the students need to develop a stronger basis in Chinese language study before they can be allowed to participate in translation. It could also be claimed that, of all the teachers here, only Dr. Liu has any cultural legitimacy to make a case for certain translations. The evidence presented here, however, shows that alongside all these disputed claims to power, or perhaps in relation with them, the translation of Chinese medicine is occurring through talk on an everyday, ongoing basis. From this perspective, power is constantly negotiated in interaction as the students resist, transform, and evoke various translation strategies from the teachers. The power, here, is not necessarily in the hands of the translator of texts, nor does it always rest in the hands of the interpreter-teacher as translator. In this interactive field, just having more knowledge does not necessarily equal having more power with regard to every participant. In the case of Dr. Liu, for example, students such as Oren and Todd have the power to demand an English translation, while other students concede to Dr. Liu's authority and attempt to learn the Chinese. Still other students, like Julia, initially resist "the crazy word" and then eventually come to realize that it is an important concept. From this vantage point, translation and power are not categories that dictate definite relations, but situated and contingent negotiations that emerge in ongoing interactions and vary among participants. Julia begins her studies with a flippant confidence about her understanding of Chinese concepts, but slowly develops an appreciation for the need to listen both to her teachers and to the Chinese language. Oren is far from convinced that such close listening is necessary, however, and staunchly refuses to forsake his quick-reference ideology of translation.

From this perspective, the co-constructed nature of most translations in Chinese medicine becomes apparent. First, we learn about the social meanings of translation in a field where everyday participants openly discuss variable evidence for translations with the intention of finding terms that work for or resonate with the way they will use Chinese medicine in their lives as practitioners. Second, we witness the extent to which participation and authority in Chinese medicine actually *require* an articulated stance on translation, how the specific demands of the field as it is currently organized in the United States necessitate participants' involvement, even as novices, in the translation of terms. Finally, the present chapter offers a set of cases in which day-to-day interaction serves as the cultural grounds for the translation of specific Chinese medical terms in the real lives of American students. In other words, we witness translation as not only a linguistic process but also an encounter between humans. These humans are vying for power in an uneven playing field and are using translation and translation talk as a social positioning tool. They are also using it as a tool of socialization into various notions of evidence and ideologies of language. With this, they participate in much larger social structures and relations of power. From this data, it becomes possible to imagine how whole institutions of Chinese medicine in the United States are often founded on translations that themselves are rooted in moral or language ideological conflicts, culturally shaped interpretative attempts to find common ground, and efforts to establish personal and cultural authority in an uncertain field. The study of translation talk in Chinese medicine thus provides a unique vantage point on the ways in which translation work unfolds in everyday interaction.

Notes

1. As noted above, Kaptchuk explains *qi* as "matter on the verge of becoming energy" (2000: 43). In the extract, Carter draws upon this commonly cited translation by saying that *qi* is somewhere "between matter and non-matter" without directly crediting Kaptchuk.

CHAPTER 5

Embodied Experience in the Living Translation of Chinese Medicine

I hold the herb and feel it, and look at it—not with hard eyes, like you know, what color is it, what's it's shape, blah blah blah blah blah. But more with soft eyes so that it's just coming into me. There's an image of it that is planting itself somewhere? And then the name—um, I will say it so that my mouth gets used to making the sounds, but I really need to let it echo in the back of my mind while I'm deeply contemplating the object. And if I do that, and that's my sole focus, and I'm calm while I'm doing it, there comes a moment where I feel in my body that I know what that is. I know what to call that.

—Treavor, second-year Chinese medical student

In this chapter, I examine the "embodied experience" phase of living translation. By showing several ethnographic examples of how specific Chinese terms are interpreted and learned vis-à-vis embodied experience, I demonstrate how embodiment, which some claim can be understood as the "existential ground" of language in general (Csordas 1994), is also the existential ground of living translation. In offering these examples, I demonstrate translation as an extended process by which meanings of terms and concepts are transmitted and transformed across cultural and linguistic boundaries. From morally and socially motivated choices made in inscription to dialogues that occur about such textual expressions, living translation in this chapter is continued in the realm of embodied experience.

Throughout this book, I have repeatedly shown teachers, translators, and students looking toward the category of experience to translate Chinese medical language into English. By experience, here, I mean the clinical experience of famous physicians in the past, the professional experience of American and European translators and teachers in their contemporary practices, and the experience of the "energy" of *qi* in the body. Although experience is, officially, a legitimate basis for truth claims in Chinese medicine (Farquhar 1994; Lei

2002), there is, we have seen, great disagreement over which types of (and whose) experience constitutes a valid basis for the translation of Chinese medicine into English. When it comes to personal or embodied experience, especially, there are ongoing tensions between scholars and practitioners (and of course scholar-practitioners) who argue about the very foundations of knowledge in healing practices. Here, the categories of "intuitive knowledge" versus "textbook knowledge" or "intellectual knowledge" are often diametrically opposed in an ontological categorization of language, and text, as against experience (Ho 2004; Van Hoy 2010). We have seen this tension emerge, especially, in the translation debates, where several participants struggle against an ideology of language that pits scholars against practitioners and argues that practitioners primarily need to develop their skills through experience rather than intellectual study.

I have shown that these kinds of tensions are embedded in the political and social history of Western language and philosophy, as well as in the history of Chinese medicine. Deeply rooted in Western ideologies where language is considered to be arbitrary, it is also tied up in the positioning of Chinese medicine as a spiritually oriented form of healing practice that offers deep self-insight. In the classroom, then, there often emerges a common ethical sensibility that favors experiential, felt learning over an intellectual engagement associated with language. One of the major ways students learn Chinese medical concepts thus involves an active embodied search for meaning or resonance, and students and teachers both often overtly emphasize a "somatic mode of attention" (Csordas 2002: 244) in their acquisition of Chinese medical concepts. Other bodies are always included in this process, invoked through discussion or literally felt in exercises that are designed to assess or treat discomfort. The self-as-experienced is also intimately involved with this learning process, especially as students search for a way of doing Chinese medicine that draws upon the deep, authentic selves of practitioners to treat equally deep imbalances of the self in patients. This is not merely an arbitrary learning strategy. It is a deeply moral commitment, as much to self or future patients as to developing the "new medicine." But even as this apparently obvious separation between language and embodied, personal experience is performed into being through exercises that are meant to distance students from abstract definitions and obscure terminology, the entire process nevertheless occurs within the medium of language and interaction and always leads back to language as words and ways of speaking come to take on meaning. This reveals that living translation, which we have already seen develop as an ongoing conversation involving multiple texts, authors, and teacher-interpreters, includes an embodied engagement as well, a journey that occurs among and within the experiential selves of participants.

Embodied experience and felt encounters with other bodies are thus key components structuring the ongoing sense-making activity that is living translation. Gadamer's notion of "coming to an understanding" as a "fusion of horizons" (2004 [1975]) provides a theoretical framework within which this embodied aspect of translation can be approached. In Gadamer's view, understanding is an event, a hermeneutic activity that occurs through dialogue and emerges as participants, each of whom arrives with a complex life-world and a host of "prejudices," develop a shared world in a conversation that simultaneously transforms and creates meaning. Although Gadamer's perspective lacks a distinct emphasis on the body as a major process, I pair his notion of understanding as a discursively emergent activity here with the notion of language as a "surging forth of embodiment" (Csordas 2002: 4; see also Merleau-Ponty 1962). It therefore becomes possible to see understanding as contingent upon language as an "intercorporeal encounter" (Csordas 2008) in which interaction is firmly rooted in embodied engagement.

This view on translation is based heavily on phenomenological approaches in anthropology and philosophy that have resisted the separation of language, embodiment, and the self, and have firmly rooted language in embodied experiences of being-in-the-world:

> Merleau-Ponty (1962) sees at the root of speech a verbal gesture with immanent meaning, as against a notion of speech as a representation of thought. In this view, speech is coterminous with thought, and we possess words in terms of their articulatory and acoustic style as one of the possible uses of our bodies. Speech does not express or represent thought, since thought is for the most part inchoate until it is spoken (or written). Instead, speech is an act or phonetic gesture in which one takes up an existential position in the world (Csordas 2002: 75–76).

Such a view presents a major challenge to the popular notion of language as somehow distinct *from* or referential *to* experience, a notion that has tended to impede the development of a theory of translation that is able to account for both language and experience. Wikan, for example, argues that in understanding someone from another linguistic or cultural community, language is simply a "ballast" (Wikan 1992: 470). In this sense, translation rests upon shared, embodied understanding that emerges over time and only partially depends on language, if at all. Similarly, Emad argues that the translation of acupuncture into American contexts involves a type of embodied translation that she deems "cultural" as opposed to "lingual" (in press).

While both Wikan and Emad embrace the notion of the embodied self as a participant in the translation process, they tend to shy away from the connection that this form of "resonance" or "transformation" has with language, either in interaction or in terms of specific words. Shifting away from the notion of language as referential form, however, reveals language as a key mediator of the embodied flow of interaction (Ochs 2010). A series of scholars have recently shown this by focusing on interaction, highlighting the role of language in the socialization of embodied habitus, including emotion and psychopathology (Capps and Ochs 1995), prayer and spirituality (Capps and Ochs 2002; Csordas 2009), and moral responsibility (Csordas 2009; Ochs and Izquierdo 2009). Such work is complemented by the abundance of scholarship in psychological anthropology and beyond that draws attention to the ways in which embodied experience mediates the learning of culture, including language (Rogoff 1995; Yafeh 2007).

In this chapter, I argue that the body and the self can also be seen as the major mediums through which language is translated as students form a working relationship with the concepts of Chinese medicine. For U.S. English-speaking students learning Chinese medicine, this means that distinct terms and ways of speaking are understood vis-à-vis embodied explanations that occur in and through ongoing interactions. Such interaction emerges not only because the students are learning specifically about the body, illness, and healing, but also because they are constantly learning in a highly intimate manner how to listen and use their own bodies to diagnose and treat other bodies through palpation, needling, and massage. This everyday practical engagement with their own and others' bodies leads them to adopt the language of Chinese medicine as their own in the sense that Bakhtin refers to as "appropriation" (1981). Prior to this appropriation, the words do not "belong" to the students. It is through embodied learning, occurring in and as conversation with teachers, texts, and peers, as well as through engagement with objects, that the words become their own. Through these interactions, they develop a "sense" of the word, in Vygotskian terms (Vygotsky 2004; as cited in Holland 1998), literally populating it with their own embodied intentions and actions. By embedding vocabulary within dialogic worlds, speakers effectively accomplish the living translation of specific terms.

Below, I offer three examples showing how embodied experience, in concert with interaction, serves as the means for making sense of specific Chinese terms, concepts, and fashions of speaking. The first example shows Treavor, in his first year, learning how to make his own sense of the translations for *po* offered in his official texts, developing his own embodied sense of the term over time through interaction. The second set of examples shows a group of first-year students grappling with the obscure language of pulse diagnosis, learning through teacher-directed activities how to translate pulse terminology into felt understanding. The final example demonstrates how one second-year student copes with the inconsistent and potentially confusing language of herb function, relying on embodied engagement with substances to understand and differentiate the words used to describe the actions of herbs. In each of these examples, felt experience, rooted in the body-self and emerging through interaction, is the existential ground upon which terms are understood by students and translated into practice. Such translations are not necessarily the most accurate representations of the meanings of terms as they are used in Chinese contexts, often reinscribing a "domestic remainder" on the term (Venuti 2000). These inscriptions are often compounded by the lack of Chinese study and the absence of clear and consistent translations in required English texts. As the examples below reveal, however, the role of embodied learning in the translation of Chinese medicine into English is nevertheless persistent and prevalent and has a great deal to offer the anthropological understanding of the relationship between interaction, embodiment, and translation.

Learning the Self

In the first example, I show how one first-year student, Treavor, takes up the struggle of interpreting *po* for himself. The *po,* as we recall from chapter 3, is translated as "corporeal soul" in most required texts. As "corporeal soul," the *po* is depicted as an aspect of the soul that is very much embodied, giving humans the ability to feel and perceive themselves and their surroundings. Alternative translations—"animal soul", "vigor," or "wits,"—are available as well, but Treavor has not yet been exposed to many of these in his first year. He struggles first with "corporeal soul." For Treavor, the linking of "body" and "soul" is a tough leap. Raised a strict Catholic, the meanings associated with the terms "corporeal" and "soul" for Treavor are opposites ripe with the indexical connotations of "physical" and "ethereal." The terms are thereby inconsistent and make sense only in opposition:

> And we get taught that *po* means corporeal soul. Those words? Don't actually mean anything. ((laughs)) Corporeal soul. Does it mean a *soul* that is corporeal? Well, that's internally inconsistent, right? ((laughs))

The translations of *po* as presented by the texts that he has seen so far in his less than one year as a student are insufficient for Treavor to understand the term such that he can use it in his own practice and own self-understanding. The explanation he has heard from other unidentified expert sources, however, proves more useful:

> Um, and uh, so when I've heard people say things like that's the aspect of your *spirit* that gives you the greatest connection to the physical *world* right, when you like, when you feel a *drive,* a drive to eat, a drive to have *sex,* like that impetus? Is the *po* speaking in you? I—*that* sinks in and then *po* stops being "corporeal soul" in my body, and it becomes that feeling, you know. So when I use the word *po* I think, this is the part of me that wants to grab and latch onto something.

Here, we see Treavor, who has been struggling with the textbook translation that he "gets taught" in class, developing a distinctly visceral understanding of the term in and through his interaction with "people" in the community. These crucial interactions, which define *po* as "that aspect of your spirit that gives you the greatest connection to the physical world" resonate with Treavor and literally "sink" into his own embodied experience. At the moment that this sinking in occurs, *po* is retranslated. For Treavor, it stops being "corporeal soul" and instead is translated directly into a felt sensation of that part of him "that wants to grab and latch on to something."

This segment offers an example of embodied dialogism in action. The indexical meanings that the words "corporeal" and "soul" have for Treavor, for example, at first prevent him from fully understanding the official, textbook translation that he is given. These constitute what Gadamer might call his distinct prejudices when it comes time for understanding to occur. In this case, they stand in the way of clear comprehension. However, through conversations he has with other experts, many of whom have probably been exposed to the alternative translations presented in chapter 3, Treavor begins to get a better sense of the term. It is only when Treavor maps or inscribes this sense onto his own embodied experience of wanting to grab and latch onto something, however, that the term really begins to have meaning for him. The translation of the term *po* thus takes on a personal, experiential component in Treavor's world that would never have evolved without interaction with—listening to—alternative sources who, with their explanations coupled with his experience, allow him to engage actively and viscerally with the term. In this sense, Treavor's process demonstrates living translation as an ongoing series of encounters through which meaning is translated in embodied moments of self-understanding that by their very nature are interdiscursive with multiple texts and multiple experts.

Learning the Pulse

The next set of examples derives from a first year, second-quarter class in which a teacher is guiding students to diagnose patients based on the feeling of the pulse. In Chinese medicine, the pulse is one of the major access points that practitioners have to patients' bodies. An adept practitioner feels the pulse for up to a minute, judging pulse length, size, rate, and rhythm to ascertain the state of a patient's bodily condition, including their organ health as well as the strength of their illness or disharmony. This comprehensive diagnostic use extends far beyond the utilization of the pulse in biomedicine, where there is a simple focus on pulse rate as an expression of timing of the heartbeat. In Chinese medicine, the pulse is felt primarily at both wrists, where the doctor places his or her fingers upon six different points, three on each wrist, each associated with specific organs. Each separate pulse is felt at three or more depths and is also evaluated in concert with each of the other pulses. This complex process yields a "pulse image" or 脉象 *mai xiang,* that is usually a composite of a number of commonly recognized pulse qualities. A pulse can therefore be said to be "floating and rapid in the lung position" or "slippery and weak in the spleen position," descriptions that suggest certain diagnoses when evaluated in concert with other signs and symptoms. The total number of pulse qualities is quite large, but some of the most common include 浮 *fu (*floating), 沉 *chen* (deep), 弱 *ruo* (weak), 迟 *chi* (slow), 数 *shu* (rapid), 滑 *hua* (slippery), 实 *shi* (replete or full), 虚 *xu* (empty or vacuous), 长 *chang* (long), 弦 *xian* (string-like or wiry), and 短 *duan* (short). Each of these includes a complex description and meaning that is often quite picturesque and somewhat opaque. "Tactile perception is notoriously difficult to put into words," writes Hsu, "and in Chinese pulse diagnosis has been conveyed in metaphors and similes, compound words and single-syllabic static verbs" (2010: 8). The words describing pulse in Chinese medicine, Kuriyama further emphasizes, "shape, at the same time as they label, what the fingers feel" (1999: 64). "Besides using different words," he continues, "diagnosticians in China and Europe *used words differently.*" A slippery pulse, for example, is described as "pearls rolling in a dish" or "small fish swimming" (Wiseman and Ellis 1996: 119). It can be a sign of either pregnancy, phlegm, food accumulation, or an abundance of *qi* and blood, depending on the copresent signs and symptoms (Wiseman and Ellis 1996: 119). A wiry or bowstring pulse, on the other hand, is described as "like a bow string about to shoot an arrow" (Li 1985: 85) or like the string of a guitar or other musical instrument (Maciocia 2005; Wiseman and Ellis 1996). A wiry pulse usually indicates a disorder of the liver-gallbladder system, but can also be associated with pain or excess phlegm.

In the Chinese medicine school in which I conducted research, it is critical for students to learn how to "read" or interpret pulses. For U.S. students, who are highly motivated to reach and affect patients' deep, authentic, interior selves, pulse interpretation becomes even more crucial for accessing, and affecting, the core truth of a patient's condition. As Barbara, the first-year diagnosis teacher seen below, states, "Patients can lie, but the body never does. Patients can be confused, but you get your hands on them and you'll find out what you need to know." In this mapping of the body, pulse diagnosis becomes "a privileged practice for bringing the appearance, the felt-sense of depth, into being" (Van Hoy 2010: 104). Students must learn how to access this depth, in themselves and others, such that they are able to proceed with treatment efficiently and effectively. To do so, they must cultivate a certain embodied sensitivity that is often, as discussed above, posited as distinct from the intellectual understanding of language as presented in texts.

In the following excerpt, Barbara is teaching second-quarter students how to feel pulses for the first time. The students are seated directly across the tables from their partners, and they are about to switch roles as doctor and patient, as Barbara designates them. Barbara calls attention to their leg positioning in relation to each other, asking them to make sure that their legs are uncrossed, "but close enough to the table that you don't have to reach to take the pulse." This means, she explains, that some students will have to position their legs such that one partner's knees are spread wide to encompass the other partner's legs or they are alternating. The class giggles with slight discomfort, but Barbara encourages them, moving her own body to demonstrate her point:

> Barbara: Get yourself in a position where there's *intimacy* here. ((undulates her hips and draws her hands toward her repeatedly)) Because that's what we're going to be dealing with now. This is a very *intimate* process. ((walks the length of the room)) Make sure your backs are straight ((turns around and stands up straight)). You know the position you take when you meditate? That's where you want to be=you want to make sure that your pelvis is tilted, ((tips her pelvis up, making a tipping motion with her hands)) that your spine is aligned, ((places one hand behind back and draws the other in a pointed motion up her center)) that there's that little string coming up from the top of your head at Du20[1] holding *everything* in line. ((dangles her pointed fingers above her head)) Your shoulders are *dropped.* ((walks back, turns, and visibly drops shoulders))

In this segment, Barbara gives detailed instructions to the students about how to position their bodies, telling them, and demonstrating with her own body, how to place their backs, shoulders, and pelvises. With her instructions as well as her demonstrations, she guides them into an intimate embodied engagement with one another. She further uses distinct Chinese medical images of the body, namely "that little string coming up from the top of your head at Du20 holding everything in line," to convey a detailed picture of how she wants their bodies to be aligned. Du20 or 百会 *bai hui* (hundred meetings) is a point located at the vertex of the head where *yang,* the active, light aspect of body and universe, is thought to converge. The name of the point derives from the understanding that "hundred" in Chinese refers simply to "many," and thus the point is where many channels converge (Ellis, Wiseman, and Boss 1989: 344). One ancient text further claims that the point "is the meeting place of the hundred spirits" (Ellis, Wiseman, and Boss 1989: 344). The point is therefore a common focus in Daoist meditations and exercises, a fact that Barbara references with her image of the string and her assumption that all of the students take a similar position while meditating. In emphasizing this point, Barbara sets up the pulse-taking exercise as a meditation as well as an intimate and embodied confrontation wherein the students must cultivate a deep knowing of their own bodies in space to read another person's pulse.

From here, Barbara leads the students through several deep breaths, groaning as she does to encourage similar bodily expression from them. They join in, and with their eyes still closed, Barbara instructs them to slide their fingers down their partner's arms to place them on the wrist. "You're going to have your fingers on that wrist for about two or three minutes," she says, "and during that time, I want you to think about two things." The first thing to think about, she continues, is "what that pulse feels like":

> Barbara: Don't worry about the words in the book. ((waves hands outward slowly and repeatedly)) We're not talking about wiry, we're not talking about slippery, we're not talking deep, we're not talking about superficial. ((continues to wave hands outwards, walks the length of room)) What we're talking about is it feels like Tigger, bouncing along. ((makes rapid bouncing motion with both hands)) Feels like water bubbling up out of a stream. ((lifts one cupped hand up in front of her as she walks)) Feels like a guitar string. It feels like a, ah, an angry bee. Just get a description of what it is you're feeling.

In this segment, Barbara is encouraging students to form their own impressions of the pulse, divorcing them from the specific words in the book. In urging them to find their own words to describe the pulse, Barbara is asking students to generate a unique language based on a cultivated learning how to listen to their embodied assessment of the pulse. It is a language of direct expression that resonates with many students in the class (see Wilce 2011). Her examples, including "Tigger," "an angry bee," and a "guitar string," are culturally familiar items that, she suggests, the students might be able to identify with physically, more than the more esoteric descriptions in the book. This physical and social positioning is key, even as Barbara invokes all of the book terms that "we're not talking about." In this sense, Barbara is using the notion of direct perception to distance the students from the words in the book, although the fact that their main text also translates a 弦脉 *xian mai* (string-like or wiry pulse) as "like a guitar string" demonstrates that Barbara's tactics actually serve to enrich the official language of the pulse by repositioning students as the generators of this very language.

Barbara continues to encourage students to focus on their embodied experience of the pulse when she further asks them to think about "not just what you feel in the pulse, but also how *you feel in your body.*" Barbara then asks students to be prepared to describe their own phenomenological experience during the exercise. She offers them several examples, telling them that they might describe an increasing or decreasing agitation and discomfort as they feel the pulse, or they might describe a specific pain in their neck or feeling of inadequacy. Regardless of what they feel, however, Barbara emphasizes the importance of attending to their embodied experience. "I want you to pay attention to what's going on in your body," she says, "because you cannot tell what's going on in someone's body until you can differentiate *what's yours* and *what's theirs.*" With this statement, Barbara promotes the notion of learning how to listen both to oneself and to one's partner within the interconnected dyad of "doctor" and "patient." Once this interconnectedness, which she terms a "circuit," is built in the intimate, embodied exchange, all kinds of feelings, both physical and emotional, can bubble over from one body to the next, creating a fusion of energies that is difficult to peel apart without a constant self-monitoring and self-awareness. In another teacher's words, this energetic back-and-forth that develops as the practitioner feels the patient's pulse can be understood as a "conversation" felt and experienced, at least initially, as wordless. To learn how to listen to this conversation is a key part of becoming a practitioner.

In Barbara's class, she guides the students into an embodied and self-focused exercise of taking the pulse. Her objective, clearly stated above, is to get them, through this close attention and intuitive listening to embodied experience, to generate their own language of the pulse and to develop a certain kind of self-consciousness in the process. In this sense, the language of their conversation about the pulse is first a culturally and phenomenologically generated language of the body. If not an entirely new language, this process makes the vocabulary in texts come alive with felt significance. To understand pulse terms in this context means merging them with self-aware, embodied experience. It means being able to name, on one's own, amorphous sensations of connection with another body. In her listing of all the terms that "we're not talking about," however, Barbara reminds students that there is an official language to eventually find one's way back to.

A continuous dance between the self-generated language of experience and the official language of the texts is therefore performed into being through an exercise intended to help students develop a felt relationship to meaning in their diagnostic practice. The next excerpt demonstrates how one student choreographs this, expertly navigating the perceived distance between experience and language. It is in the same class where Barbara is first teaching pulse diagnosis and takes place once the students have just completed their first few rounds of pulse-taking. In this context, they are each given a moment to talk about their experiences. Laura, a student, describes how her own experience of taking several pulses led her back to the words in the book that she had trouble understanding before:

Laura: But I also (.)—you know, when you read that book=and you can't figure out=I was trying to take my own pulse and I said well I don't (.4) see any difference ((places hand on her own pulse)) in the descriptives.

Barbara: Yeah
Laura: And when I was taking the pulses of the different people ((turns back to look at her partner)) I could finally realize, well maybe this does feel like a guitar string=maybe this does have those descriptives, that word in the book I could never figure out why—
Barbara: Well, that's why I don't start with the words
Laura: Right.
Barbara: Because the words get in the way

For this student, the "descriptives" in the book do not make sense when she feels her own pulse at home. When feeling pulses in class, however, she begins to make sense of some of the translations in the text. The embodied class exercise thus offers Laura a revelation, an eye-opening experience where language that never made sense before suddenly merges with her experience, coming alive in the process. Within this fusion, she begins to be able to differentiate certain pulses, saying that "maybe it does feel like a guitar string." Her choice of this particular description is notable, especially because prior to the first pulse exercise, Barbara used "guitar string" as an example that might be generated from the student's own experience of the pulse, separated from the book translation of a *xian mai* as like a guitar string (Maciocia 2005). The fact that Laura begins to feel a strong identification with the sensation of a "guitar string" pulse, however, not only corroborates Barbara's perspective that "the words get in the way," but it also confirms for both Barbara and Laura, as well as the other students listening, that the experience often does lead back to the words in the book. Barbara interrupts Laura to make this precise point:

Barbara: You know, when you can drop the words out of it and just be present to what's happening=and use your own words to describe it then you have a chance of making sense of that other stuff. So yeah.
Laura: It clarified things.
Barbara: That's a good thing to learn.

In this segment, Barbara explicitly states her conviction that "dropping the words out of it" or removing oneself from the official language of the texts is the first step in a process that includes becoming present, finding your own words, and eventually making sense of the words in the book. In Barbara's class, then, students' embodied, active learning experience becomes a site for understanding the nuances of the pulse, an occasion for the merging of official and embodied language and the creation of a space for self-knowledge to bloom. In this sense, the language of the pulse literally becomes part of the students' "bodily equipment" (Merleau-Ponty 2006 [1962]: 210) as they cultivate a certain embodied sense of ownership of the material. This "appropriation" (Bakhtin 1981; Rogoff 1995) occurs as an ongoing communicative event in which pulse terms become so much a "part of the doctor," as Barbara explains, that over time and feeling many pulses, the students will be able immediately to apprehend a person's physical condition from merely feeling the pulse. The students here learn to associate bodily experience with words and verbal expressions that critically impact the way such expressions are translated.

In these examples, I have shown how students are instructed to pay attention to their embodied experiences to understand the obscure language of pulse diagnosis in Chinese medicine. The explanation and understanding of such Chinese medical terms involves a "fusion of horizons" (Gadamer 2004 [1975]) in which language, and therefore meaning, are made one's own through embodied experience. This happens in interaction as students are socialized into the specific terms of Chinese medicine. In terms of living translation, worlds of meaning linked to specific terms are created in an embodied dialogue that occurs through the medium of hand to wrist contact. The "initial" acts of translation that occur in texts are therefore enriched as terminology becomes embedded thusly within speakers' worlds. It is only once Laura feels it to be true that the translation of *xian mai* as a "like a guitar string" takes hold for her in a form that constitutes an act of understanding through meaningful translation.

Learning Medicinals

The canon of Chinese medicinals includes thousands of substances, mostly plant-based but also including animal parts and some minerals, all generally referred to as "herbs" in English.[2] These substances are prescribed to patients based on their diagnostic profile. In cold conditions, warming herbs or other medicinals are given. In hot conditions, cooling herbs or other medicinals are given. In conditions of repletion or excess, dispersing or down-bearing substances are given, and in conditions of weakness or vacuity, nourishing or "tonifying" substances are given. Within these general categories, specific substances are chosen based on the distinct trajectory of each. So, for example, for pathologies in the spleen, substances that are understood to "go to the spleen channel" are prescribed. Each substance thus has distinct "properties," including temperature and trajectory as well as specific function. 人参 *Ren shen* (ginseng), for example, is considered sweet, slightly bitter, and slightly warm, and it enters the lung and spleen channels. Its functions include the "tonification" of the vital substance *qi,* as well as "strengthening" of the spleen and "tonification" of the lungs, among other things (Bensky and Gamble 1993: 314). Students, for the most part, have to memorize all of these properties and functions for hundreds of herbs and other products. Not only are they tested repeatedly on such details throughout the course of their study, but they need to know them intimately for clinical practice as they combine herbs and other substances into formulas for patient consumption.

Throughout this text, I have discussed the ways in which a lack of standardization has led to an overall inconsistency among texts that translate Chinese terms differently. This also commonly occurs within single texts as authors use terms inconsistently. Particularly when students do not have access to original terms in Chinese, this can generate confusion. One case in which this often occurs is with the differentiation of the terms *tonifcation* and *nourishment,* both used to describe herbs and other substances that benefit aspects of the body. Presumably, *tonify* is a translation for the Chinese term 补 *bu,* also translated as *supplement* (Wiseman and Feng 1998). As an English language neologism, *tonify* likely derives from the use of the term "herbal tonic" to describe traditional Western formulas that tonify specific organs and bodily functions. *Nourish,* on the other hand, is a translation for the Chinese term 养 *yang.* Whereas some sources underscore the fact that nourishment is distinct from supplementation or tonification in the sense that supplementation "restores strength" and nourishment "enriches and moistens" (Wiseman and Feng 1998), the main text on medicinals used in the school does not make this distinction explicit. When it comes to learning when to prescribe herbs and other substances that are described as tonifying or nourishing, then, students often ask about the differences between these actions. Julia describes how the issue emerges in her second-year herbs class:

> In here, we're talking in English, and we're getting these translations that are like kind of haphazard. They're *not* fully consistent, and so—and we get very caught up in that, and like, oh, what is *nourish*? And what is *tonify*? And duh duh duh duh.

Here, Julia notes the "haphazard" translation of terms in their texts, at first not referring to any particular set of terms. As an example, she brings up the distinction between nourish and tonify, extending this with "duh duh duh duh" to indicate that these are not the only terms where this confusion arises. Julia goes on to describe how her teacher, Lisa, a Euro-American who reportedly understands some Chinese, addresses this problem:

> And like, Lisa says these are different in Chinese concepts, but like, for your purposes in learning this right now, like don't worry so much about oh, does this one nourish or does this one tonify?

Using quoted speech, Julia explains that although Lisa does acknowledge that they are different in Chinese, she tells them not to worry about those differences for their present purposes. Instead, she encourages them to engage with the substances themselves, literally eating them, prescribing them, and watching what happens when they are ingested:

> Like understand the energetics of the herbs, and that will be clear to you. Like, it's *not* about focusing on, like, those—on the words of that. Which I understand, makes sense to me, you know. Like you learn the herb, you, you know, develop—after some time, you use the herb, you see how the herb is in the formulas, and you see what kinds of things you use it for, and you're like *OKAY,* I understand. This herb nourishes. Like I get that. Whatever.

In this excerpt, Julia is explaining how meaning is apprehended directly, through engagement with "the energetics" of a specific substance. Even for a teacher who does speak some Chinese, and could presumably explain the distinction between 养 *yang* (nourish) and 补 *bu* (tonify/supplement), this embodied engagement is the preferred strategy for connecting students to core meanings. Embodied connections with herbs and other substances are used as a tool for dealing with inconsistent and confusing translations, turning the difference between nourishment and tonification into a felt distinction, an embodied energetic. In terms of living translation, the meaning of the terms *yang* and *bu,* translated inconsistently in the texts, are translated into the dialogic world of English-speaking users as they engage directly in an embodied conversation with substances over time, with other bodies as they see the substances working and with other texts as they see them included in various formulas. The translated language of herbs, as with pulse terms, thus emerges directly out of embodied interaction, and it is only after this ongoing embodied interaction continues for some time that translated terms really begin to make sense. Although it would be desirable in some sense for a strict learning of the Chinese medical system also to require students to learn the distinctions of the terms as they are used in Chinese, this embodied aspect of translation is essential, occurring despite inaccuracies of translations at the level of their required texts.

Discussion and Conclusion

In this chapter, through a series of examples showing translation as accomplished in interactions that hinge upon embodied engagement with meaning, I show living translation to be an "interactional achievement" (Schegloff 1995) or a "fusion of horizons" (Gadamer 2004 [1975]) in which embodiment serves as the "existential ground" (Csordas 1994) for understanding. This fusion is ongoing, occurring in moments of reflection as well as action, and always involving objects—other bodies and other materials, including herbs and medicinals, texts, and acupuncture needles. The encounters within which living translation takes place can therefore be conceived of as "intercorporeal" in the sense that, as noted in Csordas (2008: 119), "being embodied is never a private affair, but is always already mediated by our continual interactions with other human and nonhuman bodies" (Weiss 1999: 5). Meaningful language that emerges out of such encounters, in this case the translated language of self, pulse terms, and herb functions is likewise intercorporeal, lodged deeply within the embodied habitus and dialogic worlds of U.S. Chinese medical students. As with all the other phases of living translation described in this book, it is a phase deeply mediated by historical and institutional frameworks, moral ideals, objects, and ideologies of language and translation.

Within this ongoing process, multiple threads of meaning are teased out and transformed into embodied sensations that never entirely overlap with the technical sense of the terms in contemporary or historical Chinese contexts. In this way, embodied translation indeed constitutes the writing of a "domestic remainder" upon the language of Chinese medicine (Venuti 2000). Such a remainder infuses the terms, whether kept in Chinese like *qi* or *po* or translated like *wiry* or *tonify,* with a felt sense of meaning, a thoroughly embodied appropriation (Bakhtin 1981) that remakes the foreign into the familiar. This kind of appropriation, especially when it is enacted with an overt disregard for distinctions made in Chinese, is arguably not the most equitable way to accomplish the translation of Chinese medicine. This inequity is amplified when participants do not learn enough Chinese to have a balanced sense of a term in its original informational context and dialogic circumstances (see Unschuld 2009; Wiseman 2000d) or when, as with Julia in Lisa's class, they are directly discouraged from doing so.

Even if students are required to learn more Chinese, however, I argue that the embodied engagement with terms will (and should) persist. In fact, engagement with the felt sense of meaning may even increase as students work to digest the historical and cultural significance of specific terms (see Goodwin 1997). This is not necessarily a bad thing. Lo (2009), for example, describes the emerging trend toward a distinct sensory approach to medical history where "capturing shared memories of odours, sounds, sensations, that surface in moments of stillness and recognition, permits recovery of something of the qualities of the past" (2009: 296). While she acknowledges the problem created by the fact that "different people sense, hear, feel, taste or see the same stimulus differently," she continues to say that "at the same time, every act of translation, of rendering the past, involves an assumption of familiarity upon which we base our interpretations. And thus the sensory turn increases intimacy" (2009: 295). This intimacy, Lo claims, can bring an interpreter closer to the text than can other methods that attempt a more critical and distancing objectivity. In Chinese medicine and elsewhere, she continues, it also opens up the possibility of establishing a more equal relationship with "the manuscript, its various authors, editors, scribes, and of course, readers and practitioners" (2009: 296). In the living translation of Chinese medicine in the field of American schools, this argument suggests that the sensual experience of participants may present an opportunity for active cultivation of a truly embodied form of listening, a relationship that deepens living translation in the long run.

Notes

1. An acupuncture point at the crown of the head.
2. The designation of all Chinese medical substances as "herbs" may be related to what Unschuld (2009) recognizes as a misguided perception among U.S. students that Chinese medicine is always natural and innocuous.

CHAPTER

6

Living Translation in and into Practice

Well, there's a new level [of translation now that I'm in practice], of course. Because, um, there's, there's the original texts. I mean, if you're talking about written texts, there are the original texts in Chinese ... There's a translation process to get that stuff into English. Within the process of teaching, there's a translation process, where teachers are helping students understand what the English language texts mean, and now I have a new job, which is I need to translate what I'm doing to my patients in a way that they can understand. And so I'm finding that, um, there is a level of specificity to which the world of academia aspires in the translation process, which is a lot loftier than the level of specificity to which I aspire when I'm trying to translate stuff for my patient. So I am often, you know, spleen stuff—you know, spleen this, spleen that—whenever the patient says to me, well, what is all this business about the spleen? I just say it's your digestive system. You know, like I can't—there's no point in trying to be more detailed than that ... [But] in order to know how—in order to know how to sort of do a broad brushstroke translation for the patient? You have to know all of the details academically, to make sure that you're within bounds. You know?

—Treavor, third-year Chinese medical student

Throughout this book, I have shown how the search for resonance in U.S. Chinese medicine emerges in the living translation of texts and practices. Apparent in inscriptions, conversations, and moments of embodied engagement, this search for resonance weaves together morally situated desires for authenticity with culturally grounded notions of healing in everyday practices of reading, writing, and teaching about Chinese medicine. In this chapter, I further show how the living translation of Chinese medicine carries forth in the practice of acupuncture, herbal prescription, and the pursuit of effective treatments that are resonant with patients' conditions. In a very basic sense, this translation emerges in everyday moments of communicative engagement where interns or practitioners translate Chinese medical terms for patients. These are the moments when the sense of participation examined in the inscription, interaction, and embodiment phases of living translation becomes real, where the practitioner "does translation" as a core part of her job. Part performance, part patient socialization, translation in practice is an important opportunity for interns and practitioners to assert their authority, build rapport with patients, and start generating clinical results. In a second sense, the living translation of Chinese medicine also emerges in the moments where the language students have learned through their long journey of reading, listening, evaluating, embodying, and communicating comes together in the diagnosis and treatment of patients. As the culminating achievement of all their years of study, the translational moment where "theory" becomes "practice" is what is really at stake for most of the participants in this study.

This chapter looks at both kinds of translation, showing how translation emerges both *in* and *into* practice as part of the living translation of Chinese medicine. In both cases, translation arises at the intersection of learning and action, embodied understanding and communicative effect. Moments of translating for and "upon" patients thus serve as a critical site for further investigating the multiple tensions implicated in the translation of Chinese medicine into English, tensions between authentic historical understandings and authenticating practices (Pordié 2012; Van Hoy 2010), between biomedicine and CAM, and between so-call "scholars" and "practitioners." These are moments where we can directly witness translation becoming further entangled in multiple cultural representations, complex relationships with biomedicine, and public desires for difference.

Theoretically, this chapter continues to incorporate a distinct focus on co-construction, viewing interaction with patients and about patients as part of the process of living translation. In this sense, engagement with patients, both in language and in action, are "zones of encounter" (Zhan 2009) in which the translation of Chinese medicine is collaboratively constructed in an ongoing stream of communicative activity. At the very center of this interaction, there is the need to develop rapport and establish authority through both verbal and nonverbal communication (see Heritage and Maynard 2006). This often begins with the "simple" translation of Chinese concepts, including *qi*, *yin*, *yang*, or *po*, for patients. In American contexts, the "other" of such translations and explanations is commonly assumed to be biomedicine, and very often the intern needs to learn how to translate Chinese medical language to patients using the common ground of the biomedical body. In one sense, this serves the purpose of basic explanation in terms that the patient will understand. In another, it establishes the practitioner as a medical authority conversant with biomedical language (Katz 2011). At the same time, practitioners need to ground their explanations in a clear presentation of how Chinese medicine differs from biomedicine, especially because many Chinese medical patients have little to no experience with acupuncture or herbal medicine (Cassidy

1998a). They come, however, because they are inspired by the idea of a holistic model of medical care, either on the basis of personal ideologies or negative experiences with biomedicine (Cassidy 1998a). Practitioners are thus often forced to act as cultural translators for their patients, at least in their initial visits (Emad 1998; Katz 2011). What ends up happening is that acupuncturists "find themselves challenged to translate-create alternative metaphors for an alternative-hungry clientele or readership" (Emad 1998: 44). In translating for patients, then, practitioners must walk a thin line between biomedicine and alternative medicine or CAM, commonality and difference. They must draw together these multiple ways of thinking about illness and the body at the same time as they enact their differences through language. This takes "coordination" as Mol calls it, referring to the process by which "varying realities ... are balanced, added up, subtracted ... [and] fused into a composite whole" (2002: 70). In the present case, this coordination emerges partially as a constant negotiation of multiple meanings in interaction with patients. Just like in the classroom, such interactions are ongoing and, as Treavor's statement above suggest, involve multiple participants, including texts, teachers, peers, and the patients themselves, in an encounter where the practitioner is now placed in the role of interpreter or "language broker" (Garcia-Sanchez and Orellana 2006). Within this context, the practitioner must establish, as with any author or teacher, her authority to translate.

There is more at stake than merely legitimation strategies in translating for patients, however. The process of aligning with patients is also a key part of the initial and ongoing healing practice that is Chinese medicine in the United States. This alignment, Kaptchuk reminds us, "can resonate with the condition ... and induce a person toward health" (Kaptchuk 2000: 46). A connection with the person one is needling is thus a crucial part of the healing relationship (Zhuo 2007: 386). Although it might seem from certain angles that this connection is purely "physical," students are constantly reminded of the importance of language in the building of rapport with patients. Language, in this configuration, is the foundation of resonance, the ballast that lets the well-placed needles resound in the patient's body. Students hear about it from their textbooks and their teachers, where they are constantly reminded that it matters how they talk to their patients, the way they explain things to them, and the way they translate concepts for them. Even before I began my own studies in Chinese medicine, for example, a speaker at a school open house told the group that our future success would critically depend on the way we learned to talk about Chinese medicine, the way we would translate it for potential patients. At a recent lecture for licensed practitioners of Chinese medicine, one well-regarded speaker reminded the audience that patients "hold on" to what they (we) say to them both diagnostically and by way of explanation. She said this instructionally, to remind listeners to take care to frame their diagnoses and prognoses positively to help them emerge from the state of being "unwell." Practitioners of Chinese medicine are thus very aware that they must "do things with words" when they are working with patients (Austin 1955).

Language, in this sense, is a critical part of what might be termed "patient socialization" (Stivers 2012), a process linked to treatment effectiveness in that it not only directly impacts the treatment dynamic, but it also helps the patient reframe their experience as "transformative":

> Such terms as "meridian," "qi," "Wind cold treatment," and "energy" and words describing the patient's state of health, such as "deficiency" and "excessive *Yin*" characterize the treatment and the patient's health in accord with a Chinese definition of the body, health, and therapy. The accordant invocation of Chinese medical terminology further characterizes [the patient's] bodily responses as therapeutic sensations and not simply as painful. Other word choices ("arise," "deep," and "rest") signal that a transformation is occurring in [the patient's] body, and hence, in her state of health (Anderson 2010: 262).

Language, in this case the use of Chinese medical terms in interaction with the patient, serves the purpose of creating a harmonious experience, itself a crucial part of the resonance that is required for true transformation and healing to occur. In this sense, the language used in the clinic becomes a site for the effectiveness of treatment as well as the expression of difference and the establishing of legitimacy. It is also an opportunity for practitioners to demonstrate their professional ethic of care, using language to align themselves with a holistic, patient-centered model that intentionally focuses on aspects of the spiritual, emotional, and environmental self.

Observing and considering language behavior in practice is therefore a rich site for examining multiple aspects of the living translation of Chinese medicine. Translation *into* practice is also, however, an opportunity to observe the living translation of concepts like *jing*, *qi*, *po*, or, as above, "wind-cold." In this sense, the formulation of treatment strategies can itself be understood as a kind of translation. As Karchmer (2004) observes about Judith Farquhar's research on Chinese medicine in practice:

> Her work demonstrates that *bianzheng lunzhi* [diagnosis of pattern and determining of treatment] can be thought of as a method of translation, a strategy for transforming the clinical presentation of the patient into the therapeutic intervention of the physician. As with translation, the "target language" of the prescription—usually a collection of herbs or a set of acupuncture points to be needled—should reflect as fully as possible the "source language" of the clinical presentation (Karchmer 2004: 154).

Translation in this sense is akin to the currently popular "translational medicine" that focuses on translating basic science discoveries and research outcomes into clinical care, also referred to as "bench to bedside" (Goldblatt 2010). This constitutes the translational moment when diseases, and cures, are enacted. This is a simple translation in neither Chinese medicine nor in biomedicine. As Mol (2002) describes, even in biomedicine, "if we no longer presume 'disease' to be a universal object hidden under *the* body's skin, but make the praxiographic shift to studying bodies and diseases while they are being enacted in daily ... practices, multiplication follows" (2002: 83). The act of creating interventions further "enact an object by altering it" (2002: 89). To alter the object, the body, or illness as it is enacted through multiple interpretations in Chinese medicine, practitioners must draw upon years of textual study, embodied practice, conversations, and lectures. This is the anticipated moment in which "book knowledge" merges with "experience" to yield a honed intuition or intention (Farquhar 1994; Karchmer 2004). The role of language in this translation has yet to be deeply examined, however, in either biomedical or Chinese medical contexts.

This chapter thus seeks to address both translation in and into practice in contemporary U.S. Chinese medical education. Although ideally this inquiry would be grounded in ethnographic observation of intern-patient interactions in the school clinic, I was unable to secure ethical clearance at my field site to observe clinical encounters. Throughout my fieldwork, however, I was able to observe several key participants move from being first- and second-year students learning in the classroom to being observers and finally interns in the clinic. I was also able to observe and video-record several case-review courses, in which third- and fourth-year interns discuss real clinic cases anonymously in a group format. This chapter is therefore based on a combination of classroom observation, participant interviews, and video recordings of case-review sessions. The first section examines one particular student's development of a distinct interactional style in the translation of bodily organ terms for patients. The second section focuses on translation into practice through the analysis of one classroom example of a case discussion where interns, with their supervisor, co-formulate a treatment plan for a single patient whom they determine is suffering from a form of post-traumatic stress disorder (PTSD). In both sections, we see the practice stage of living translation in the school as it is enacted through translating for and upon patients.

"Kidneys But Not Really Kidneys": Living Translation in Practice

In this section, I look at the translation of internal organ terms in Chinese medicine to examine how translation in practice emerges in conjunction with social, historical, and political translation choices as well as personal and cultural ideologies of health and healing. As I discuss briefly in chapter 1, the Chinese medical body consists of five chief organs, translated consistently across multiple contexts as the heart, spleen, lungs, kidneys, and liver. There is a great deal of discussion within the school and other Chinese medical communities about the use of these Western anatomical terms to translate the names for the Chinese organs, however. In the most popular texts on Chinese medicine, for example, the fundamental differences between Chinese and biomedical organs are stressed. Maciocia thus writes that "when studying the Chinese theory of the Internal Organs, it is best to rid oneself of the Western concept of internal organs entirely" (2005: 97). Kaptchuk (2000) similarly states, when discussing the organs, that "Chinese medicine is a coherent system of thought that does not require validation by the West as an intellectual construct" (2000: 77). In these formulations, there are two separate bodies posited, one "Eastern," one "Western."

In this two-body system, the Western body is pictured as "structural," and the Eastern body is depicted as "functional," directly mirroring the late-nineteenth-, early-twentieth-century construction of the structure-function dichotomy, which Karchmer explains "preserves essential differences" at the same time as it constructs the two bodies as "mutually complementary" (2004: 89). For example, while the Western medical heart is considered an organ in the thorax responsible for pumping blood through the organism, the Chinese medical 心 *xin*/heart is responsible for "housing" the mind, or *shen,* and "opening" to the tongue in terms of taste and speech, among other things. The spleen, or 脾 *pi,* an organ of blood storage and lymphocyte production in biomedicine, is a central digestive organ in Chinese medicine. In this sense, the spleen is said to govern "transformation and transportation," referring to the transformation of food and water, as well as the distribution of *qi* and blood derived from nourishment. Because of this, the spleen is said to work in close conjunction with the stomach. The 肺 *fei,* or lungs, in Chinese medicine regulate the waterways and are seen to connect with the skin and large intestine, among other things. The 肾 *shen,* or kidneys, are responsible for growth, development, and reproduction, as well as connecting to the bones, brain marrow, lower back, and ears. The 肝 *gan,* or liver, in Chinese medicine is responsible for ensuring the smooth flow of *qi,* including emotions, throughout the body, among other things. The liver also "stores" blood, governs the sinews, and is connected to the eyes and nails. Within each of these definitions, the many roles that are common to both biomedical and Chinese medical organs, such as the heart's job of pumping blood, the lung's role in respiration, the kidneys' role in urination and water metabolism, and the liver's involvement with bile, as well as the common locations and structures of the organs in each system, are deemphasized. For this reason, some translators have argued for the use of distinct terms to designate the Chinese organs, including "orbs" (Porkert 1974) or at the very least the use of capital letters to differentiate Spleen from spleen, for example, as we saw with Maciocia in chapter 3, as a deployment of the orthographic resource of capitalization to encode an imagined semantic difference.

This entirely different body, in many ways, fits with the expectations of the students, who are studying Chinese medicine to learn something different than biomedicine. At the same time, it is unclear how exactly to relate the two. In this regard, several seemingly contradictory statements are made in the texts. Maciocia thus writes that "whereas Chinese medicine excels in its acute and detailed observation of complex functional relationships, it does not entirely disregard the study of anatomy" (2005: 97–98). Right after telling readers that the Chinese medical body needs to be approached as an entirely different entity than the anatomical body of Western medicine, however, Maciocia proceeds to suggest that there are indeed many instances in both classical and modern Chinese medical texts in which the anatomical structures as at least physically understood by biomedicine are clearly described. In his text, moreover, the orthographic differentiation between "Organs" versus "organs" is not always deployed consistently, blurring the proposed difference between the two. Chen (2005) likewise explains that the theory of the organs in Chinese medicine was developed through ancient anatomical knowledge, claiming that the practice of anatomical dissection in China actually predated the practice in the West (2005: 28). While this is a historically problematic claim, there is nevertheless widespread acknowledgement within the scholarly Chinese medical community that the organs translated as heart, spleen, lungs, kidneys, and liver do now and indeed have always referred to the same anatomical structures identified by biomedicine (Hsu 1999; Unschuld 1985, 1998; Wiseman 2000c).

In terms of translation, Wiseman therefore dubs the use of alternative or capitalized terms to designate the Chinese medical organs as "semantically deviant" and claims that it belies a distinct form of discriminatory practice:

> Chinese medicine does accord functions to the internal organs that differ from those that Western medicine accords them. This is not surprising, since its original authors did not have the technology to detect the microscopic structures and understand the biochemical reactions upon which the modern understanding of the organs is based. Nevertheless, this is a matter of understanding how the organs work, not a matter of identifying them. The semantically deviant translations effectively reformulate traditional Chinese concepts simply to accommodate the modern medical understanding. Ultimately, they merely serve to assert the Western medicine understanding of the body as the true understanding, and distort the original Chinese conception (Wiseman 2000c: 247).

In emphasizing the commonalities between the Chinese medical and Western medical bodies, Wiseman argues against the kinds of translations that create totalizing difference where there actually exists much more overlap in understanding.

Wiseman here exposes the inherent ambiguity and deeply embedded social politics in the structure-function dichotomy that posits two separate Chinese medical and biomedical bodies. Recalling the discussion in chapter 1, the structure-function dichotomy was historically crafted as a legitimation strategy to defend Chinese medicine against the dominance of biomedicine in the late nineteenth and early twentieth centuries in China (Karchmer 2004). In this formulation, then, the ever-present "anatomy-problem," described by Karchmer, was the impetus behind efforts to "Orientalize" the Chinese medical body by restricting its sphere of understanding, and influence, to the mysterious and ineffable "functional" (Karchmer 2004) and "experiential" (Lei 2002) realms, leaving anatomical "structure" to a more physically powerful biomedicine. Wiseman thus asserts that efforts to translate Chinese medical organs with different names, when they clearly *also* belong to the same structures as recognized in biomedicine, maps the normativity of biomedicine onto the language of Chinese medicine and distorts the true basis of bodily understanding in Chinese medicine. Lo (2009: 294) further emphasizes that "[r]ather than mapping the body's functionality, many early Chinese textual and visual sources that describe the medical body portray and convey aesthetic knowledge of 'things perceptible to the senses'" (see also Lo 2001). Finally, Kuriyama (1999) points out that even in Western medicine, especially historically, the organs were seen as centers of "activity" much more so than merely structures (1999: 263). From this perspective, the structure-function dichotomy is seen as a distinctly contemporary, economically, and politically motivated interpretation of Chinese medicine.

In the contemporary United States, the normativity of the split between the biomedical body and the Chinese medical body is nevertheless preserved, even though the organs are generally referred to with biomedical anatomical terms in clinical and classroom settings. As demonstrated in the last chapter, students constantly use their own bodies as an experiential basis with which to mediate their understanding of the language used to talk about this ambiguous and multifaceted body or set of bodies. This is not only an embodied engagement with the language, but a moral one as well, a judgment about which body is better to think with or to heal with. In conversation with patients, however, the fact that biomedical organ terms are used so broadly in Chinese medicine remains a central concern, especially because there do not seem to be any hard and fast rules about how to explain the true difference.[1] Most of their patients, they are often reminded, will come to them with distinctly Western notions of the organs, and they will be forced to translate the language they use into terms patients will understand. To find a way to do so without creating unease or confusion is a top priority. In the following clip, the students are in their first-quarter Fundamentals course. It is the third week, and Carter, their instructor, discusses the impact that Chinese medical organ terminology often has on patients:

Carter: In a TCM clinic, they'll feel your pulse and they'll say "Oh yeah, heart pulse is weak," and then the patient will say, "My *heart*? But is my heart okay?" You know, because we said, oh, heart pulse is weak=but course we mean all these other things, right? But the patient doesn't know that. They haven't taken this class and four years of study.

In this segment, Carter begins by designating TCM practitioners, deictically referenced as "they," as using a language reflective of a different ontology of the body than the patient. "Heart pulse is weak," a phrase that "they'll" say, is thus meant to index the functional heart in TCM. The patient, however, interprets the reference to "heart" as denoting the anatomical heart of biomedicine. Here, Carter uses what Agha (2007) calls "represented speech" to position the practitioner and patient in an ethically situated encounter in which unmediated TCM language may alarm uneducated patients, who "haven't taken this class." In effect, Carter also performatively invokes the presence and importance of the patient's voice in students' future practice. This is brought home in the subsequent lines, where the deictic reference shifts to "we," indexing the students as participants in the TCM community of practice and the ongoing tension between what practitioners say and what practitioners *mean* in the clinic.

In the following part of the interaction, Carter describes the ways in which alternative schools of practice in U.S. Chinese medicine have approached this issue. In contrast to TCM, then, Worsley practitioners, who subscribe to an alternative framework based on the five phases and developed by British practitioner J. R. Worsley, use an innovative language so that "they don't illicit a reaction from the patient," says Carter. This way, Carter explains, improper understanding of terminology will not influence "the outcome of the interaction" with the patient. Here, Carter overtly relates the language spoken in clinic to the outcome of healing, stressing the fact that certain kinds of practitioners choose an intentionally distinctive jargon, a jargon that is in fact even more functionally distant from the structural body, to avoid confusing and alarming patients. Although he is not advocating that his students learn this alternative language, especially because they will be expected to use the common translations for the organs throughout their schooling, Carter is introducing the students to a certain ethics of language behavior in the clinic. From this vantage point, students must be prepared to explain the different bodies to patients to avoid scaring them and thereby compromising treatment success. In other words, they must possess close-at-hand translations that differentiate Heart from heart, Spleen from spleen, and so on. Translation here must be more than historically accurate or culturally authentic. It must *serve* the instrumental goals of treatment.

This lesson sticks with the students. When she first becomes an observer in the clinic, for example, Julia complains about interns "throwing around" terms that could be confused for biomedical designations and not explaining them well:

> And so when someone, you know, I would see interns throwin' around like, oh, well, your spleen *qi* is just tanked, like in, you know ... And people would be like my spleen *qi*? Like what does that mean?

Julia's image here is vivid, offering us an image of strange words being thrown around casually, sparking the alarm and confusion of uneducated patients. In Julia's perspective, however, definite time constraints limit the ability of interns to explain the concepts adequately. Continuing with the example of an explanation that might follow a statement such as "your spleen *qi* is just tanked," then, Julia describes how she has witnessed certain interns attempt to translate the Chinese medical spleen to patients using language directly translated from Chinese such as "the spleen is in charge of transportation and transformation":

> And they're like well, basically the spleen is in charge of transportation and transform—and like launch into this thing, and it's like *they* don't know what you're talking about. You know, like you can't explain that to somebody in like three minutes when you're laying them down on the table for an acupuncture treatment.

For Julia, these real-world constraints on how much they are able to translate for patients gets her thinking seriously about the ethics of language in the clinic and how she wants to use communication as a tool in her own budding practice:

> It's a whole part of that *protective space*, you know? I don't want words being used that they don't understand. I mean, that's not comforting, when you hear a word and you don't understand what it means. (.) It's unnerving.

Here, Julia invokes the "protective space" that she imagines creating for her patients. For her, this involves lighting, music, atmosphere, objects, and language. In this context, obscure language seems to index a situation comparable to biomedicine, where the use of incomprehensible language is "unnerving." As a clinical observer, then, Julia is critical of interns who use detailed and confusing explanations to provide opaque or inadequate translations for patients.

Later in her own journey to becoming an intern, Julia realizes that many of the patients that come to her actually *want* to hear her speak in unfamiliar, foreign terms:

> They know that we have this other language that we learn and we speak, and they seem to be drawn to it and curious about it. That's why they came to the medicine.

Here, Julia continues to observe the way language can be drawn upon to position herself as different from biomedical practitioners, not just in the sense of creating a different kind of "space" for patients, but also in fulfilling their expectations of a different kind of jargon. At the same time, the issue of legitimacy and proving oneself conversant in the language of biomedicine also ends up playing a role in Julia's developing sense of herself as an interpreter of Chinese medical language:

> They understand Western medicine stuff better, and so it's nice when you can throw like a little—like even if you're referring to a part of the body, you know, to like throw a little Western medical terminology—it grounds it as far as patient comfort level. I mean, you know, patients are comfortable with doctors, which of course is bizarre, because doctors kill more people than anybody, but like—((laughs)) but I mean, you know, they *trust* that language.

Julia thus often "throws in" a little Western medical language, using it as, she later states, "a comfort tool" with patients to engage their sense of trust, as misguided as she judges that to be. She continues from here by explaining that when she refers to the upper arm area as the humerus, for example, patients respond positively. "They're all like ooh, she knows about the humerus, like she must know about being a doctor." Here we witness Julia learning how to handle the balance between a "foreignizing" and a "familiarizing" approach to translation, using a mixture of language patients desire and language they trust. Julia is thus learning how to position herself as an authority figure who, despite acupuncturists' status as "not quite doctors," (Katz 2011), "knows about being a doctor." In other words, she uses language to enact the body as a known scientific entity at the same time as she uses it to enact herself as an authority. Although we cannot directly witness it here, it is likely that this balance also varies among interactions with different patients, emerging in concert with a constant back-and-forth assessment of patient perception and comfort.

Translation with patients comes to involve a delicate balance of finding a language that resonates with patients as different yet understandable. This is a social skill as much as it as a social role. It is especially challenging for students who are steeped in the ambiguity of the structure-function dichotomy and in many ways are forced to develop their own explanations for how the internal organs of Chinese medicine relate specifically to the anatomical structures of biomedicine. In this sense, the inherent ambiguity in Chinese medical diagnosis (Hsu 2010) is significantly amplified by the uncertainty inherent in available translations. As Julia grows into a third-year intern, however, she learns to bridge the two more fluidly:

> I mean, the piece that I always focus on that seems to really help with that is to start by telling patients that the name—like kidneys—it does not mean your physical kidney. Like it's just a word that we use to talk about a—really, a whole *system* of things that ranges from things that we would think of as genetics, to things like water metabolism and stuff like that. And different stuff having to do with energy,

> and that even emotional stuff like fear. You know, I'll sort of throw around a bunch of examples like that, to show them that it's really this huge, wide range. I say "and so we're really talking about this whole system."

Here, Julia reveals the extent to which she identifies with the Chinese medical community, using the deictic "we" to reference the language "we use" to talk about the whole system of things that is not actually the physical kidney. There are also remnants of her personal ideology of language, expressed during her first quarter and seen throughout the present volume, where kidney happens to be "just a word" that actually refers to something other than the physical structure. Again using "we," she goes on to translate how "we would think of" the kidney system, using a circumlocution or intralingual translation to accomplish an interlingual or cross-system explanation (Jakobson 1966 [1959]). Here, she mixes a biomedical category (genetics) with Chinese medical categories of "energy" and "emotional stuff" with what could be considered a category in either system (water metabolism) to produce a translation that is both comforting and reasonably informative. After confidently "throwing around" these explanations, Julia describes, she will also explicitly discuss translation with patients, explaining that the translation "kidney" is actually not accurate:

> And I usually would say, it was poorly translated to be kidneys, which is what—the word that we use. But it does not, you know, mean—but then sometimes I'll say you know, it can have you know some correlations actually too, like for example the lower part of the back, which is obviously where these kidneys—you know, where the kidneys are, is the part of the body that is ruled by the system which I'm speaking of. So I'll, you know, I'll kinda, you know, talk to them while I'm setting them up and stuff like that, um, and I think it really helps patients?

In this part of the segment, Julia positions herself as an interpreter of both the original Chinese and the terms used to "poorly" translate those terms, although she does not, as we have seen her teachers doing, refer to the agents of such poor translations. In this sense, Julia is performing an expert metaknowledge about translation that also effectively accomplishes a specific translation. She thus explains that while she and her community of practitioners use the word kidney, it both does and does not mean exactly the same thing as the biomedical kidney. She goes on to describe it, laughing, as "kidneys but not really kidneys." This is where Julia starts to hedge a little bit around the issue, using a question form and rising intonations, perhaps indicating her uncertainty about the ways in which the correlations actually play out. Nevertheless, she relays all this to patients while she is setting them up for acupuncture, and according to her interview report, it seems to really help them.

In this section, I have shown part of Julia's journey toward becoming a practitioner, highlighting her discovery of the need to translate Chinese medicine for patients. At once capitalizing on their desire for difference but also appeasing their need for familiarity, Julia learns that translation in practice is a balancing act between proving her own legitimacy and educating patients, making them comfortable in her healing space and providing effective treatment. This is not an easy accomplishment, especially because of the history and politics embedded in most of the translations that Julia has been exposed to. This history is literally mapped into the language used to talk about the body in Chinese medical school and is repeated over and over again in the classes that Julia takes. Beginning, as we saw, in the Fundamentals class, it continues in many other contexts, where teachers continually invoke the difference between "energy medicine" and Western medicine. In this sense, the living translation of Chinese medical organ terms in the classroom and in practice tends to reproduce the inherent ambiguity in historical translations that describe the Chinese medical body as entirely different than the biomedical body, even despite the relatively consistent use of what Wiseman would term the so-called correct interlingual translations of heart, spleen, lungs, kidneys, and liver. One might even argue that the power dynamics behind the translation of Chinese medical organ terms are much bigger than the translations themselves and through discursive reproduction vis-à-vis a living translation that includes commentaries, interpretations, and patient interactions, have contributed to the blurring of the line between "true" and "false," making the structure-function dichotomy when it comes to the translation of bodily organs in contemporary U.S. practice almost entirely true. Combined with the propensity toward a separation between spiritual or mental/functional realms and physical realms in the United States, this perhaps amplifies the distinction between structure and function as it is enacted in contemporary China. While a doctor in a hospital in China may, for example, code-switch between organ terms multiple times in a single utterance, the overall effect is a strong linking between the structural and function bodies, distinct as they may be. Here, when they are retranslated into a framework of alternative medicine, there is the danger that the organs of Chinese medicine become even more detached from the physical body (Karchmer 2011, personal communication).

Translation as social action is here enacted in a social space that, similar to the early twentieth-century context in which the structure-function dichotomy was worked out, has explicit economic and political implications. In serving a social purpose, such translations achieve the same goals in the contemporary United States as the structure-function dichotomy was originally created to serve. They deproblematize the potentially destabilizing relationship between the Chinese and biomedical bodies and create a public discourse that can easily place Chinese medicine as a complementary or alternative medical practice, nonthreatening in its fundamental difference and effective in its own domain. Translations that preserve the structure-function dichotomy serve to coordinate differences. The particular danger with this distinction, especially in the context of a U.S. community that aims to transform healthcare by utilizing a holistic approach, is that Chinese medicine is increasingly pigeon-holed into a "functional" medicine without structural effects and without a precise language to describe its connection to anatomical structures.

Although this was only one student's journey, her experience suggests that each intern learns, over time and largely through actual engagement with patients, to approach translating in practice: sometimes with quick glosses that crystalize years of learning, sometimes through sputtering attempts to explain everything, and sometimes confidently sweeping over the technicalities of the relationship between the "structural" and "functional" bodies. As in other contexts, this activity is morally and ethically situated, often emerging in the process of enacting an alternative spirituality or holistic medicine, the "protective space" of CAM vis-à-vis biomedicine or in developing a reputation as a "team-player" in an integrative context. In this sense, the participation framework situating the intern and patient is at once historically and institutionally determined *and* socially emergent. "Speech participants" writes Agha, "choose referring expressions through practices that involve reading the interactional context of the moment of referring" (Agha 2007: 94). In translating for patients, this context is both emergent and firmly located in a sociohistorical frame. Although it is often broadly informed by multiple versions of the structure-function dichotomy, in many ways it is also developed anew in each interaction, contingent upon the micropolitics of engagement as well as the continuous embodied and social learning of the intern. The ongoing, inherently plural nature of this reproduction constitutes the basis for understanding living translation in practice.

Echoing into the Body: Living Translation into Practice

I had this idea in my head that when I finally got around to learning therapeutics, what I was going to discover is that these points are buttons, just like an aspirin is a button. So if, you know, if there's a particular issue, you press the button, and psshtt, you know, something happens. And now, after taking this class—it's really obvious to me that these aren't buttons that we press to have a specific effect. These are—to use language that I think you'll appreciate—these are translational devices. Acupuncture points are translational devices. I need to have a conversation with the inner workings of my patient. I don't speak spleen, right? But if I see what's going with the person, and it happens to be a spleen-related issue, I can stimulate a certain selection of points, and that particular pattern of point selection echoes into the body, and evokes a response in the body, so that the body will pay attention to something that maybe it hasn't been paying attention to. It's like hey! You need to wake up, and look at this, 'cause you're not—that's there and you're not doing anything about it, and you need

> *to do something about it. I could—I could say that to a person, but you know, their energy system isn't going to react to that. So my translational device is these points. I work on the points, and the points say, in a language that the body understands, ah, there's something happening here that we need to be paying attention to, guys, let's pay attention to it.*
>
> —Treavor, second-year Chinese medical student

As I discussed in the introduction to this chapter, translation at the intern level not only happens in interaction with patients, but also emerges as students learn to translate the language of Chinese medicine *into* practice in the crafting of diagnoses and treatment plans. As both Karchmer (2004) and Farquhar (1994) highlight, choosing the right acupuncture points as well as the right formulas can be understood as an act of translating understanding into action, enacting translation through practice. It is also a prime method of further establishing resonance with the patient, the *gan ying* that emerges in the very interaction of the needle and the patient's body (Zhuo 2007). As we can observe in Treavor's comments during his second-year experience of learning acupuncture points, this interface between practitioner and patient is embodied in a dialogue where the practitioner's intention literally echoes through the patient's body. Although it is clear here that Treavor uses the language of translation to please me—he says directly "to use a language that I think you'll appreciate"—it is also clear that the metaphor of translation serves to aptly represent Treavor's understanding of how the treatment, in many senses, unfolds as an intercorporeal conversation between practitioner and the multiple parts of the patient's body-self.

In the school where this ethnography was conducted, this kind of translation into practice could be directly witnessed both in the clinic rooms where interns were needling patients and offering them medicinal formulas, as well as in case study forums where fourth-year interns met with various clinic supervisors to discuss specific cases. The following example comes from such a forum, a "case review" session in which Barbara, the teacher we have seen repeatedly throughout this book, is helping a group of interns work out treatment strategies for a single patient. The format is the same as in other case review sessions, where a single intern presents a genuine clinic case to the room, using a relatively standard case form to summarize the chief complaint (CC), history of chief complaint (Hx CC), signs and symptoms of chief complaint (S/S CC), other signs and symptoms (Other S/S), family history (Family Hx), menses, medications, observation, palpation, blood pressure (BP), pulse, and tongue, as well as the diagnosis (Dx), treatment (Tx), and herbal prescription (Rx).[2] Chinese medical students in the contemporary United States are taught with this case form to *see* their patients' conditions according to this set of standard categories. Although the details and content may differ, there are many parallels in the way students in biomedical programs who learn over time to reorganize patients' disjointed narratives into a coherent case presentation format (Apker and Eggly 2004; Atkinson 1981, 1988; Beagan 2001; Bosk 1979; Davenport 2000; Good and Good 1981, 1993, 2000; Light 1980; Montgomery 2006; Sinclair 1997).

In this particular case review course, interns are also asked to record the patient's desires for improvement as well as the intern's intent for the patient. This is reflective of Barbara's personal and professional identity as a practitioner concerned with emotional health, patient-intern connection, and especially developing the interns' sense of themselves as practitioners. It is also a function of this class being geared toward the use of "extraordinary" channel points in devising treatments that go beyond the functions of general TCM treatments. Although in this way the review class is somewhat unique, I should also mention that it is by far the most popular case review session in this school and is highly regarded by students.

The following case study, focusing on a patient with the chief complaint of anxiety, was distributed to the classroom and then described by the treating intern. As usual, a question-and-answer period follows the case presentation in which the other interns as well as the teacher are allowed to ask multiple questions about the patient. At that point, the interns work individually or in groups of two or three to construct alternative treatment strategies. At the end of about thirty minutes, during which time Barbara circulates the room, sometimes making announcements in response to what she sees different interns working on, the class reconvenes to discuss several specific treatments. While Barbara plays the role of chief interpreter of the treatments, grilling the interns about their point choices, the entire class often participates in an animated discussion about the validity of the treatment, any problems the treatment might generate, or ways in which the treatment could be improved. Such discussions provide a unique opportunity to witness the way translation into practice emerges as an ongoing discursive formulation of the conversation that is unfolding between practitioner(s) and patient. As we shall see, this involves a constant back-and-forth to ascertain what the patient is saying, what the interns want to say back, how to say it, and where the dialogue might go from there.

Case Review Study

Female, 44
Born in Iran, divorced, no children

CC: anxiety
HX CC: Patient feels anxiety is fear based. She describes childhood as "uncertain," "anxiety ridden," and "unstable." She moved to U.S. in her

teen years. She has had anxiety since she can remember and always has felt insecure and uneasy. For 20 years she has been having severe panic attacks during which she "freaks out" often in public places and can't catch her breath so she gasps for air and gets dizzy. She has agoraphobia due to such severe anxiety and feels like she has no control in the moment. Even attending group meditation class is frightening to her as she is worried she will have a panic attack. She also has asthma which provokes anxiety.

S/S CC: palpitations, SOB, stuffy sensation in chest, unable to pull breath past diaphragm, "stuck" feeling in chest

Other S/S: History of asthma since childhood with labored breathing and difficult inhale. History of anemia. Poor circulation: cold hands and feet. Varicose veins and spider veins along SP channel. Plumpit. Acid reflux, which triggers asthma, which then triggers anxiety. Frequent sighing. Frequent yawning. Urinates 1x//night but sleeps okay otherwise. Sometimes struggles to fall asleep due to worry and anxiety. Gas and bloating after eating. Bloating is sometimes visible in her upper abdomen. BM 1x/day well formed. Thirst with aversion to ice cold drinks.

Family Hx: She is very close to her mother and brother. She is the only one in family with anxiety. Doesn't like to talk about Iran and hasn't been back since she left. She still has family there whom she doesn't keep in contact with.

Menses: Cycles getting shorter. @ 25 days. Alternating watery red and thick dark red with clots. Flow 3-4 days. Very emotional PMS.

Medications: Nexium (acid reflux)

Observation: Patient is fidgety and restless. She sighs frequently and has a difficult time breathing deep. There is a noticeable energetic separation between her UJ and MJ. Her ribs are slightly visible on her chest. Her eyes are at times struggling to adjust, and they shift from smiling to fearful. Her eyes look as if in distress and portray a deep sadness. She frequently adjusts her posture from slightly hunched to sitting straight. She is very grateful for her treatments at the clinic and often reminds me of how "wonderful" all the interns she has had are. She has made significant progress in the last 2 years and attributes all the progress to having acupuncture. She accepts no credit for the proactive work she herself has done. She wants to get over anxiety and feels desperate to break the chains that bind her.

Palpation: Her abdomen is warm, and she is slightly guarded. There is a lot of tension along her Ren channel and ST region.

Patient's wish from the treatments: To slow down the "chatter" in her head and feel calm.
My intent for the patient: To help her to pull her breath into her dan tien and connect with her feet. I want her to trust that she has control over her state of being and grasp the concept of mind over matter.

PR: 78
BP: 130/82
Pulse: wiry, thread, congested in LV position, thready in HT position
Tongue: red tip, dusky body, red sides, yellow coat

Dx: Ht and SP qi xu, LV qi yu, Damp Phlegm accumulation
Pts: HT 7, 3/ CV 22, 19, 17, 12, 6/ ST 25, 36, 40, / Sp 6/ GB 8, 40/ Yin Tang or DU 20

Rx:	*Suan zao ren 18*	*bai zhu 9*
	Chuan bei mu 9	*zhi shi 9*
	Yuan zhi 6	*Fu ling 12*
	Huang lian 3	*Dan dou chi 6*
	Gua lou 12	*xiang fu 9*
	Yu jin 6	*zhu ru 6*
	Jie geng 9	*lu gen 9*

Abbreviations: CC: chief complaint; S/S: signs and symptoms; SOB: shortness of breath; SP channel: spleen channel; Hx: history; PR: pulse rate; BP: blood pressure; ST: stomach channel; LV: liver (position on pulse); HT: heart (position on pulse); Dx: diagnosis; Ht and SP qi xu: heart and spleen *qi* deficiency or vacuity; LV qi xu: liver *qi* deficiency or vacuity; Pts: acupuncture points; Rx: prescription.

From just reviewing the case study form, the first thing that perhaps becomes apparent is the switching back and forth between multiple types of genres and perspectives to present the case. For example, several terms indexing a biomedical or psychiatric understanding of the patient, such as "panic attacks," "agoraphobia," and "anxiety," are used throughout the document. Specific Chinese medical terminology and ways of speaking are also included, for example "spider veins along SP channel" (spider veins on the spleen channel, which runs along the inside of the legs), "Plumpit" (sensation of something in the throat, short for "plumpit *qi*"), and "thirst with aversion to ice cold drinks" (a standard Chinese medical way of describing a patients' temperature and internal moisture). Likewise, the abbreviations, organization of information, and presentation of objective measures encodes a distinct medical, if not necessarily biomedical, flavor to the text. At the same time, the patient's experiential or "subjective" voice is heard strongly throughout the case, including her emotions, her physical sensations, and her desires. The clinical observations of the intern are often similarly presented in a language that further reveals her own "subjective" engagement with the case. For example, in writing that "her eyes are at times struggling to adjust, and they shift from smiling to fearful," or that "I want her to trust that she has control over her state of being," the intern indexes her multifold involvement with this patient.

This kind of involvement is expected in Chinese medicine and is actively cultivated. This is the case not just in this class, where there is a distinct focus on psycho-emotional treatment, although it is perhaps more encouraged and openly discussed here. In the average case study, interns are always balancing objective and subjective perspectives, biomedical and Chinese medical registers, and the patient's voice with their own, intersubjectively constructed voice. In this sense, they could be considered to be engaged in a kind of professionalized genre-mixing, where each intern engages in a complex conversation with the patient, translates it into a coherent presentation, and then further translates it into a set of actions that will extend the conversation in an intended direction. On the case study form, however, it is difficult to observe the process by which the intern comes to arrive at the particular points (PTS) and herbs (RX) that she needles and prescribes on the particular session that is represented in the document, which she reports have been devised in conversation with Dr. Liu, whom we heard from in chapter 4, as the supervisor. One could backtrack and derive, based on the points selected and the herbs and medicinals prescribed, that the treatment was constructed out of a translation of "heart and spleen *qi* vacuity, liver *qi* depression, and damp phlegm accumulation" into a set of actions designed to quiet the heart, supplement the spleen, course the liver *qi*, and transform phlegm. This does not necessarily offer any insight into the translational process itself, however. Observing the following classroom interaction in which multiple interns are engaged in trying to translate this complex case into a set of coherent actions thus offers the opportunity to witness the living translation of Chinese medicine into practice.

The interaction begins with the chief intern presenting the case to the class, reading from her case report but also adding certain innovative mixed-genre descriptors to depict the patient. This sometimes involves mixed-code neologisms such as, for example, "upper jiao-y," to indicate that her symptoms are located largely in the upper part of her chest, known as the "upper jiao" in Chinese medicine (上焦 *shang jiao*). The treating intern receives questions, all increasingly focused on the psychological or functional imbalance of the patient, from her peers. The first question asked comes from an intern with a background in psychology, "Has she had any treatment specifically for PTSD?" This is answered with a definite no, as the patient has not felt comfortable in psychological therapy of any kind. The questioning intern persists, however, in identifying the patient's set of symptoms as PTSD related to her childhood in Iran, which she does not like to discuss. Following questions include, among other things, whether the patient gets anxious only in public spaces, whether she tends to wear certain colored clothes, how she responds to needling, how she sleeps, whether her asthma and anxiety are connected, whether she uses an inhaler to control her asthma, and her marital status. The answers evoke a much more detailed picture of the patient's life circumstances, her appearance, her work, her emotional and embodied experience, and the methods by which she controls her symptoms. At one point, the chief intern reiterates how much she likes this patient, how "sweet" she is, and how much she would like to help her. "But I feel like I'm in a rut," the intern complains, and after a few more questions, the interns break up into groups to discuss the case and generate alternative treatments.

The following segment derives from the classroom discussion that emerges in conjunction with the sixth treatment to be discussed in the group. Prior treatments have repeatedly invoked the diagnosis of PTSD, despite the lack of official diagnosis, solidifying the group's assessment that she is suffering from a certain identifiable psychiatric condition. The discussions have further analyzed the patient's condition from many angles, translating it into multiple kinds of treatment meant to "balance the top and bottom," as well as to "deal with the emotional issues." During the course of about thirty-five minutes, the conversation between the interns and Barbara constantly translates between biomedicine and Chinese medicine, TCM and alternative approaches to Chinese medicine, and between treating this patient and treating in general. Multiple interpretive frames of reference are invoked in this interaction, including, notably, the students' texts. At one point, a popular text is problematized for listing a point function that differs from another text, and the whole room shifts their focus to their books. Barbara asserts her interpretive authority in relation to the contested text, here, saying, "I'm not really buying that," and relating her interpretation specifically to this patient. "It's hard to talk about errors because there's not a lot of textbooks that really lay out which is which," she says. Because of the more esoteric nature of the material on the extraordinary vessels, she further explains that "not all of it is written" and very few practitioners really know it all. To be safe, she suggests, interns must relate the information they derive from alternative sources with the information provided in the standard texts and weigh both when they treat patients.

Directly after this discussion of texts, the following interaction emerges. In it, the group is discussing the treatment devised by a group of two interns in order to treat PTSD and disperse accumulation in the chest.

> Barbara: Okay … with the Lung 5 and the Kidney 4, so let's look at that in terms of PTSD What's involved in that? Why does that make sense? What happens to a person when they suffer (.) trauma?

Barbara begins her interpretation of the treatment under discussion by asking the interns to look at the reasons why the acupuncture points "Lung 5" and "Kidney 4" might be indicated in PTSD.[3] From this perspective, PTSD is invoked as a distinct set of responses that transpire when a person suffers trauma. Before any of the interns can respond, however, Barbara continues by qualifying what kind of traumatic circumstances underlie the PTSD they are confronting with this particular patient:

> Barbara: And in the case of patients who've had PTSD=very often it's really a very dramatic trauma, or repeated trauma over a long period of time, right? You get one bomb going off, that's a pretty big shock. But if every day when you wake up=there are bombs going off around you, pretty soon you're gonna have PTSD.

Barbara's characterization of PTSD in the case of this patient has more to do with repeated trauma over time than any single instance. The group's historical analysis has placed her in Iran during the 1960s, when political unrest under the Shah government likely would have exposed her to a great deal of violence, including frequent bombing. Barbara here shifts the "relational centering" (Hanks 1992) of her remarks from an impersonal patient to a second person "you." With this act, she personalizes the understanding of PTSD, placing it as a simultaneously universal and specific response to repeated trauma. In response, the students translate "what's going on here" into Chinese medical terms:

> St1: Is that—so scattered *qi*? [that's involved]
> Barbara: [Yeah, what happens there?]
> St2: There's no [exhaling]
> St3: The lung *qi* is in fear. The fear affects the kidneys and then you have the lung=and you have the lung, the *wei qi* constantly (.) There to protect them [so then the kidneys are being attacked]
> Barbara: [Yeah, so that *wei qi's* being] depleted and attacked repeatedly over and over again.

Here, the interns begin to translate into technical terminology like "scattered *qi*," a possible effect of repeating violence. Barbara confirms this translation and further questions them as to the dynamics involved. While one student relates it to a lack of exhalation, another translates it into the emotional response of the lung's *qi*. She thinks on her feet here, working it out in terms of how this dynamic of scattered *qi* and persistent fear might reverberate through the body via the kidneys and the *wei qi*, or the *qi* associated with the lungs and the skin, usually translated as "defensive" or "protective" *qi*. She immediately ties the fear in with the kidneys, as fear is the emotion generally associated with the water phase that includes the kidneys and bladder. However, in the next line, the lung comes back online because of the relationship that the lungs and kidneys have in the production of *qi*. It is useful here to understand also that the kidneys are seen to "grasp" the inhaled air from the lung. As the intern is working out the details of this relationship in terms that pertain directly to this patient and more generally to the translation of PTSD, Barbara overlaps her speech and encourages an analysis involving *wei qi*, which is being depleted. Barbara then continues by invoking the *po*, the spirit of the lung that we saw many divergent explanations for in chapter 3 and that we saw Treavor struggle to make sense of in his own body in chapter 5. Here, Barbara builds her *own* translation of the *po* in a set of statements that further personalizes the *po* at the same time as translating it into biomedical terms:

> Barbara: Plus, you have the spirit of the lungs, right? The *po*=When you have that kind of trauma, that has a physical safety thing, where you have—your, your *po*'s job is to *feel* everything in a *corporeal* kind of way, right? Is to *respond* to your external environment in an *autonomic* reflexive kind of way, and if that's, um, you know, a, a *shocking* or traumatic thing, over and over and over, and over again, pretty soon the *po* says, okay, I'm outta here=checkin' out, goin' on vacation call me when this settles (.) 'Cause maybe I'll come back then, maybe I won't, right? ((interns giggle)) So there is a huge relationship between the lung and kidneys=in terms of how you respond to big kinds of stresses. Huge.

In this part of the segment, Barbara brings up the *po* as an addendum to the present discussion, invoking the corporeal aspects of the *po* by linking them to the felt experience of repeated threats to physical safety. Again, the relational centering of the *po* here involves the students, who each have a *po* themselves. "Your *po*'s job," she says, "is to *feel*," thus experientially grounding the discussion in a felt physiological response that everyone can identify with. This response is characterized as passive and interior: it responds to the external environment reflexively. Here, Barbara invokes the autonomic nervous system of biomedicine, the most non-agentive form of response. Recalling Dechar's explanation of the *po* as relating to the "primitive" structures of the autonomic nervous system, the limbic system, and the cerebellum, we can perhaps begin to locate Barbara's translation in the conversations emerging at the intersection of psycho-spiritual and biomedical interpretations of Chinese medicine.

At this point, however, she shifts back to the original characterization of PTSD and trauma, the reoccurring shock, and begins to formulate the *po* as itself an agent with its own distinctive voice. So the *po* here is "modeled through discourse" (Agha 2007: 51) as (1) having a distinguishable voice that speaks a casual genre of English, (2) having an agentive positioning, where it can just up and decide to go on vacation, and (3) is able to be reached later by telephone, but again, can still decide whether to come back or not. This modeling of the *po* elicits giggles from the students. We can imagine that if Treavor was in the class, he might be thinking about "the part of himself that wants to grab" suddenly getting up and going on vacation, trying to reconcile his own embodied construction of the *po* with the discursive construction of the *po* evidenced here. We can guess that this is in fact happening for many of the students as they giggle in response to Barbara's "translation" of the *po*'s words in a novel language that they nevertheless understand. For those who have read the many translations of *po* described in chapter 3, moreover, there is a need to make room for this distinct interpretation of what Kaptchuk calls the Animal Soul and Dechar links to deeply instinctual notions of right and wrong. At the same time, they need to reconcile the translation of *po* as autonomic nervous system, a distinctly non-agentive and reflexive response to the environment, which one cannot usually directly control.

The interaction continues with a further discussion of how the patient's asthma ties into the PTSD and how it will be addressed with this treatment. It ends with a return to discussing the clinic book, with Barbara saying that she has not checked the text to see about using this approach for the treatment of PTSD, "but that *logically* it makes sense." At the end of class, a group of interns stays behind discussing with Barbara the extent to which such an emotional involvement with patients takes a toll on their own energy. Barbara agrees, and uses the opportunity to underscore the importance of them getting regular treatments themselves.

Taken as a whole, there is an enormous amount happening in this interaction. I cannot necessarily address everything here. I want to focus, however, on the translational process and the way in which it unfolds over the space of about forty minutes of collaboration and discussion. Most prominently, it is an opportunity to observe interns developing a distinct mixed-code professional register in interaction, a "professional vision" (Goodwin 1994) that they use to translate experiential data into action. This register involves frequent code-mixing, including interspersing of Chinese terms into their discourse. It also includes a constant negotiation of biomedical and Chinese medical speech genres and the movement back and forth between different perspectives and stances. In deciding why to use a combination of the acupuncture points Lung 5 and Kidney 4, then, there is an intricate and ongoing translational process that incorporates multiple stylistic shifts. In addition, we also witness the ongoing nature of the discursive modeling of particular organs and the further reproduction of the structure-function dichotomy into a clinical assessment that focuses almost entirely on "function" vis-à-vis a contemporary biomedical psychiatric diagnosis (PTSD).[4]

The process of decision-making and action-forming in clinical interaction is not necessarily always this overtly collaborative. In certain professional contexts, including integrative clinics, professional case forums, and Internet Listserves where practitioners discuss cases and treatment strategies, it most certainly is. However, this segment suggests that, regardless of how it occurs, the process of translating Chinese medicine into practice is a deeply intersubjective and contingent process that involves multiple participants in an ongoing stream of discursive engagement. As I suggested in the last section, the patient is not removed from this stream, a body acted only upon. In Chinese medicine more than any kind of biomedicine, we can perhaps witness the incorporation of the patient's voice in practice-based translation (Emad 1998). In this sense, the patient's embodied experience regularly becomes a further site for translation as he or she responds to the treatments: squirms in reaction to certain types of needling, complains about the taste of the formula, or reports that certain configurations of points make him or her feel really good. Emad (1998) thus approaches the bodies of acupuncture patients as "translative mediums" (1998: 33) through which Chinese medicine is conveyed in the contemporary United States. In terms of the current analysis, I further suggest that the ongoing conversation with patients—the translation of their experience into action and their responses to those actions—are a key part of the "living" translation of Chinese medicine in the United States.

Discussion and Conclusion

In this chapter, I have shown that from the beginning of their program, students are taught that the way they speak matters to patients. It is not only crucial in developing trust and initiating resonance with a new patient, but it is also a key method by which students learn to establish their legitimacy as acupuncturists and herbalists vis-à-vis biomedical practitioners (Katz 2011). As described above, it is also an essential component for framing the patient's experience as therapeutic and transformative rather than painful or strange, a factor that aids the effect of treatment and further confirms the legitimacy of the practitioner specifically and the medicine more generally. For these reasons, the issue of translation emerges as a critical site for developing students' budding sense of themselves as practitioners, and serves as a key site for living translation.

With a focus on the way this process emerges in the context of the translation of organ terms, the first section of this chapter demonstrates the ways in which students and teachers participate in the ongoing dialogue through which Chinese medicine is translated in action. This dialogue is emergent in the socially contingent interactions that serve to complete the translations offered in texts and in lectures in multiple, diverse ways. It is also both historically and socially situated in a political, economic, and ethical context. In this sense, a translation strategy that was developed in the particular context of twentieth-century China has traveled through both space and time to become an accepted truth about Chinese medicine in the contemporary United States. Here, as we saw in the second part of the chapter, an intense focus on the functional amplifies the structure-function dichotomy to such an extent that one could argue that instead of creating a truly holistic approach, the Chinese medicine body becomes even more detached from the anatomical body in the United States (Karchmer 2011, personal communication).

From this vantage point, one cannot help but wonder about the ways in which translation both generates and disinhibits the practice of Chinese medicine. Would things be different if there were an official way to translate "beyond" the structure-function dichotomy? How have specific practitioners maneuvered around it in their various ways of explaining the organs to patients? What would a more "authentic" translation look like? Again, these are complex questions that, at this stage, can benefit from a view of living translation as it unfolds at this specific historical moment in the United States. In combination with similar studies observing the multiplex enactment of structure-function translations in practice in China (Karchmer 2010, Scheid 2002), it demonstrates the ways in which translation can be a site for both creative resistance, as well as for perpetuating complex relations of power between a dominant biomedicine and alternative forms of practice.

In this chapter, I have also shown how living translation emerges *into* practice in the context of diagnosis, prognosis, and the development of specific treatments. Here, translation is a complex activity that involves, as in other classroom contexts, multiple "voices" (Bakhtin 1981, 1986) that are jointly used to translate the experience of the patient, the experience of the intern, the definitions in texts, and the wisdom of the teacher in a deeply heteroglossic conversation that further contributes to the modeling, through language, of both terminology and meaning in Chinese medicine. Expert voices are prominent at this level of translation, but equally contributive are students' own embodied understandings as well as the embodied and spoken responses of patients. At this point, it is as much a learning to *speak* as it is a learning to listen.

In both situations, the living translation of Chinese medicine unfolds as a discursive, embodied, social, moral, political, and economic engagement that further extends the inscriptions, interactions, and embodied experience that I have examined in the last several chapters. Living translation does not end here, of course. Inherent in the living nature of the process, it continues throughout the interns' lives as they formulate their own practice, interact with more patients, continue their reading, attend conferences, and write manuscripts. For the purposes of the present study, however, the tracing of translation from text to practice in the everyday lives of American students concludes with this view on living translation as an engagement with and for patients.

Notes

1. See Hsu (1999: 206–210) for a discussion of the difficulties inherent in trying to find a precise terminology that captures the difference, but also preserves the structural integrity of the Chinese medical body.
2. See Andrews (2001), Karchmer (2010), Scheid (2002), and Taylor (2001) for a detailed history of the historical development of the case study format in Chinese medicine, especially the adoption of a biomedical style of presentation.
3. Lung 5, or "cubit marsh," is located on the crease of the elbow, lateral to the biceps tendon. Generally used to treat conditions of lung heat (cough with or without blood, chest pain, asthma) and phlegm as well as in some stomach conditions (vomiting, diarrhea), it is also used to regulate lung *qi* or *wei qi* (Deadman and Al-Khafaji 2001; Jacob 1996). Kidney 4, or "large goblet," is located on the inner ankle just next to the Achilles tendon. It is used to treat conditions like fear, back pain, poor memory, and depression, among other things (Deadman and Al-Khafaji 2001). Jacob (1996) also lists the point function for Kidney 4, when used in combination with Lung 5, as "Lung post traumatic stress" (1996: 137).
4. Although not part of the current study, it would be interesting to conduct a cross-cultural examination of the ways in which Chinese interns performed the translation of a similar case. Research has suggested that such "psychologizing" or "functionalizing" of illness along the lines of generating deep self-growth is considerably less prominent in China (Zhang 2007), and Karchmer (2011) suggests that this type of complete "floating away" from the physical body would never occur in a Chinese case study room (personal communication).

Conclusion

Learning to Listen

> *The currents of tradition that are Chinese medicine thus do not merely refer to a genealogy of concepts, but also to the networks through which these concepts are transmitted from the past to the present.*
>
> —Volker Scheid, Currents of Tradition in Chinese Medicine

In this text, I have elaborated upon the notion of living translation as an ongoing stream of personal, social, and cultural activity, a process of contentious debate, of searching for resonance, of creative inscription, of interaction with texts and teachers, peers and patients, as well as an embodied, self-oriented experience of language learning. A process of practice. Visible in the multiple, deeply felt tensions between CAM and biomedicine, classical Chinese medicine and TCM, language and experience, living translation emerges in inscriptions in texts as well as in classroom contexts where teachers use translation talk to position themselves as authorities with regards to information originating in a different language and time. It also emerges in the responses of students to their books, their sensorimotor and emotional involvement with the texts as well as their ongoing dialogue with teachers and patients. Living translation is likewise woven together in the composite pieces of the ongoing terminology debates and, as I showed in the last chapter, has a direct impact on translation in everyday practice. All of these phases, I hope to have successfully conveyed, are always deeply intertwined and overlapping.

In this grand multiplicity, living translation is inherently uneven and fundamentally diverse. History lives in the language emerging out of living translation, often, as with the structure-function dichotomy in early-twentieth-century China, creating effects that can actually confound participants' greatest efforts to translate a "new" kind of holistic medicine. Power and politics are not far behind history in shaping the way institutional practices of prioritizing biomedical classes over Chinese history or language study influence the way living translation is enacted in everyday worlds. These institutions, or more specifically the diverse sets of teachers within each institution, generally guide students toward attuning to different aspects of Chinese medicine, but often such guidance is resisted. That resistance, for better or for worse, is also part of living translation and can only really be appreciated through an ethnographic analysis of the micropolitics that often structure interactions within and outside of the institution.

All of this together leads to certain quantifiable, but also qualitatively measurable transformations. Most prominently, there are transformations in language that emerge out of a combination of all of the translations together—*po* becomes "corporeal soul" (Wiseman and Feng 1998) as well as "Animal Soul" (Kaptchuk 2000), the force most related to the thyroid hormones thyroxine (T4) and triiodonthyronine (T3) (Kendall 2002: 124), "a force that draws things in toward the center of our being and holds them there" (Jarrett 1998: 260). The *po* further becomes the part of Treavor that wants to grab and latch on, but for students working with the translation of PTSD in Barbara's class, it is also the autonomic nervous system and a part of the self that can get up and go on holiday when it is afraid. *Qi* becomes both "energy" and "not-energy." It is a feeling of heat in the ankle, an indexical of the "new medicine," and a concept that is just too difficult to translate accurately. *Yin* is rheum, or mucus, or a "phlegmy-but-not-phlegmy" snot-like substance. Within all of these translations, the meanings of the terms are made and remade, formed and transformed through inscriptions, interactions, embodied experiences, and practices that are quite successful in mapping a "domestic remainder" (Venuti 2000: 485) of meaning and value onto the Chinese terms at the same time as they transmit basic information. All of these living translations are moreover heavily mediated by institutional and historical realities, moral frameworks, material goods, and ideologies of language and translation.

Transformations are not limited to language, however. In the context of the present study, students continuously and very consciously involve their deepest selves in the process of learning Chinese medicine, including especially the language to use with patients and with which to talk about patients. This process occurs over time, occasioning a deep and ongoing transformation in self-perception and techniques of self-care. As Julia states in her second quarter, "I mean, the medicine is so real, and just like, it just speaks to the truth in a way that, like, you cannot help but look at yourself." Treavor, as well, experiences Chinese medicine as a radical reawakening, effected in large part through new ways of thinking and speaking about himself, of a part of himself he thought he had permanently lost. In this sense, living translation provides an opportunity for personal as well as linguistic transformation. Not limited to the private realm, it is also a transformation of the professional self, as students become practitioners. In both of these cases, transformations in ways of being and ways of seeing arise out of ongoing conversations that translate, interlingually and intralingually as well as intersemiotically, the living language of Chinese medicine.

Finally, institutional transformations issue forth from the process of living translation. The translation of Chinese medicine as a science, for example, has given rise to institutions in both China and the United States that draw upon a textbook-based, classroom format. Although this does not necessarily completely transform the everyday practices of Chinese medicine at the level of individual physicians and teachers, it does participate in the continuation of translations that work to create a comfortable bedfellow for biomedicine out of Chinese medicine, rather than resisting such integration. In the United States, the translation of Chinese medicine is still very much contested, and various institutions are in competition for the rights to define the language of the profession. In the ensuing debates, both institutions and language are transformed.

If one accepts all of these transformations as part of the lived process of translation, then it becomes clear that some amount of change is impossible to avoid. Where, then, does that leave the arguments of scholars and practitioners who suggest that "to transmit Chinese medical knowledge to the West, we must translate, not reinvent" (Wiseman 2002b: 22)? The basis of these arguments, we have seen, is largely cultural and vastly moral. At its root, it is about having respect for a deeply textual tradition with a highly developed language that deserves to be translated accurately. From any vantage point, this argument is important in attuning us to the dangerous clinical and social effects of translations that blindly transform traditional concepts, especially when such transformations evolve out of interactions between people who have never studied Chinese.

Here, however, I would like to again pick up the strands of resonance, listening, and relationship introduced at the outset of this text. As I have shown throughout this study, learning the language of Chinese medicine is a long process of searching for resonance—in texts, in the classroom, in the clinic room, and in relationship to oneself. This living translation is a multifaceted conversation with many factors to consider. Not only a search for equivalent words, it is a search for authority, legitimacy, interpersonal authenticity, and clinical effectiveness. In any single conversation, one can thus view multiple priorities and power relations in negotiation. Living translation is therefore not just doubly hermeneutic, as Gadamer might suggest. It is, in fact, multiply hermeneutic and often shifting.

The multiplicity of living translation complicates the seemingly simple dichotomies between East and West, traditional and contemporary, scholarship and practice that are commonly drawn upon in ideologies of translation that focus solely on word meaning or on cultural politics. It also challenges theories of translation that, in their insistence on viewing source and target cultures as binary, tend to obscure the inherent dialogism in emergent processes of translation. Such theories, I hope to have shown, alert us to the many problematic implications of transformation when it comes to translation, effects that can and do have far-reaching consequences. To access the vitality of translation as a living process, however, I hope also to have shown the importance of focusing on relationships, on the blurred boundaries between texts and practices, the institutional representations of language and the embodied understanding of meaning. This opens up the space for reevaluating ways in which a *dialogic* view on translation in which participants actually learn how to listen to multiple voices, including the voices of the past, of original authors, as well as teachers, patients, and the voice of their own embodied experience can help the field of Chinese medicine move more toward the collaborative cultivation of translations and transformations that resonate with more than just a single voice or one-sided cultural perspective.

In this sense, in this book, I hope also to have shown that the study of translation as a living process does not necessarily mean uncritically accepting the uneven relations of power that often structure translation, nor does it mean turning a blind eye to the specific architecture of intersubjectivity or the anatomy of intertextuality in Chinese medicine. If anything, such a view demands a well-constructed theoretical framework to apprehend the multiple, ongoing processes of transformation that together comprise the core of living translation. For this, I have relied upon a collection of theories and methodological approaches, including especially sociolinguistic and discourse analytic notions of co-construction, indexicality, and action-in-interaction; phenomenological understandings of inscription, reading, and learning; as well as critical studies of the relationships between institutions and individuals. I have shown the many ways in which moral notions of healing and self-awareness and growth, material artifacts such as texts and even acupuncture needles, ideological notions of what language is, and institutional practices of science and education consistently influence the multidimensional process of living translation.

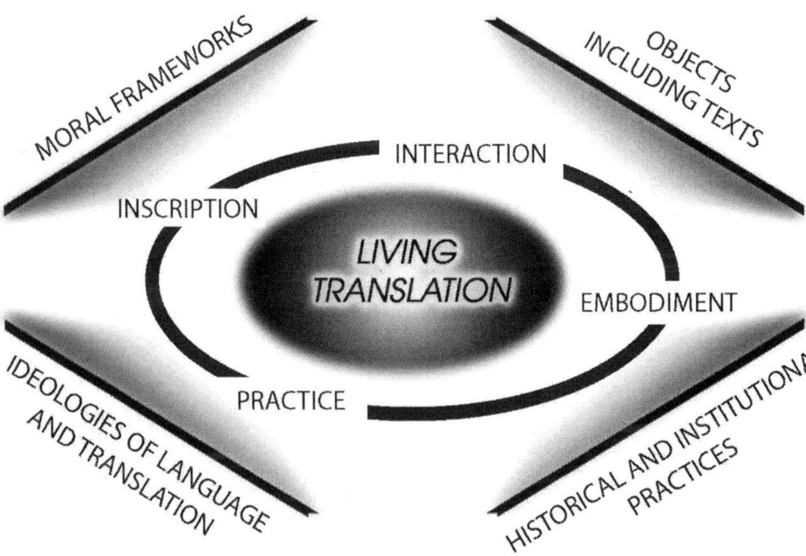

In this sense, I hope to have created a tentative model for the emerging anthropology of translation that understands translation to be a deeply human process with multiple actors and multiple effects. Given that I also subscribe to the view that any anthropological inquiry is always also an intervention of sorts (Scheid 2011, personal communication), it is my hope that the ethnographic story of living translation presented here can further contribute something toward healing the divide between "scholarship" and "practice" at the level of language in the translation of Chinese medicine in the United States. I envision the intervention in this particular case as an encouragement of sorts, a recognition that while increased communication with Chinese sources is necessary, embodied engagement with language and conscious reflection upon the ways in which Chinese medicine is translated in everyday interaction is also critical. In this sense, I advocate for the development of a certain kind of awareness in professional Chinese medicine (call it "anthropological," if you will) of the ways in which history, culture, morality, and variable notions of personhood shape the way we all, myself included, participate in living translation.

Although the concept of living translation grew out of a particular ethnographic situation, it need not necessarily be limited to describing this context. Particularly in the translation of health practices, including but not limited to yoga, martial arts, meditation, Ayurveda, and various forms of integrative medicine, living translation offers an analytical lens that allows for the simultaneous appreciation of broad cultural processes, everyday interaction and practice, writing and reading, embodied experience, and moral notions of personhood. As a model or roadmap for constructing ongoing ethnographic studies of socialization in medical anthropology and beyond, it also provides a foundational effort toward understanding how people, practices, and meanings change over time. In this broad sense, this study aims to participate in recent efforts within anthropology to create cross-subfield dialogue between sociocultural, linguistic, medical, and psychological anthropology. In my own small way, with living translation I also hope to further the interdisciplinary relationship between anthropology, medicine, philosophy, history, and translation studies in the construction of the anthropology of translation as a distinct and vigorous field. I firmly believe that it is only with such cross-disciplinary conversation that we can productively address the complexities of contemporary experiences in translation.

References

Abel, Jonathan E. 2005. "Translation as Community: The Opacity of Modernizations of *Genji monogatari*." In *Nation, Language, and the Ethics of Translation*, ed. Sandra Berman and Michael Wood. Princeton and Oxford: Princeton University Press, 146–158.

Abu-Lughod, Lila. 1991. "Writing Against Culture." In *Recapturing Anthropology: Working in the Present*, ed. Richard G. Fox. Santa Fe: School of American Research Press, 137–162.

Agha, Asif. 2007. *Language and Social Relations*. Cambridge: Cambridge University Press.

Aikhenvald, Alexandra. 2004. *Evidentiality*. Oxford: Oxford University Press.

Anderson, Kevin Taylor. 2010. "Holistic Medicine Not 'Torture': Performing Acupuncture in Galway, Ireland." *Medical Anthropology* 29, no. 3: 253–277.

Anderson, R. 1976. "Perspectives on the Role of the Interpreter." In *Translation: Applications and Research*, ed. Richard W. Brislin. New York: Gardner Press, 208–228.

Andrews, Bridie. 1996. "The Making of Modern Chinese Medicine, 1895–1937." Ph.D. dissertation, Department of History, Cambridge University.

———. 2001. "From Case-Records to Case Histories: The Modernisation of a Chinese Medical Genre." In *Innovation in Chinese Medicine*, ed. Elisabeth Hsu. Cambridge: Cambridge University Press, 324–341.

Anelo, Carmen Guarddon. 2005. "Philosophy, Anthropology and Linguistics in Translation." *Translation Theory*. Available: http://www.proz.com/translation-articles/authors/70/Carmen-Guarddon-Anelo,-Ph.D./ui, accessed November 15, 2008.

Apker, Julie, and Susan Eggly. 2004. "Communicating Professional Identity in Medical Socialization: Considering the Ideological Discourse of Morning Report." *Qualitative Health Research* 14, no. 3: 411–429.

Appadurai, Arjun. 1996. *Modernity At Large: Cultural Dimensions of Globalization*. Minneapolis: University of Minnesota Press.

Appiah, Kwame. 2000 [1993]. "Thick Translation." In *The Translation Studies Reader*, ed. Lawrence Venuti. London and New York: Routledge, 417–429.

Aravamudan, Srinivas. 2006. *Guru English: South Asian Religion in a Cosmopolitan Language*. Princeton, NJ: Princeton University Press.

Asad, Talal. 1986. "The Concept of Translation in British Social Anthropology." In *Writing Culture: The Poetics and Politics of Ethnography*, ed. James Clifford and George E. Marcus. Berkeley: University of California Press, 141–164.

Atkinson, Paul. 1981. *The Clinical Experience: The Construction and Reconstruction of Medical Reality*. Franborough: Gower.

———. 1988. "Discourse, Descriptions and Diagnoses: Reproducing Normal Medicine." In *Biomedicine Examined*, ed. Margaret Lock and Deborah R. Gordon. Dordrecht: Kluwer, 179–204.

Austin, J. L. 1955. *How to do Things with Words.* Cambridge, MA: Harvard University Press.

Baer, Hans. 1995. "Medical Pluralism in the United States: A Review." *Medical Anthropology Quarterly* 9, no. 4: 493–502.

———. 2001. *Biomedicine and Alternative Healing Systems in America.* Madison: The University of Wisconsin Press.

———. 2004. *Toward an Integrative Medicine.* Walnut Creek: Alta Mira Press.

Baer, Hans, et al. 1998. "The Holistic Health Movement in the San Francisco Bay Area: Some Preliminary Observations." *Social Science and Medicine* 47: 1495–1501.

Barcan, Ruth. 2011. *Complementary and Alternative Medicine: Bodies, Therapies, Senses.* Oxford and New York: Berg.

Bakhtin, Mikhail M. 1981. *The Dialogic Imagination.* Caryl Emerson and Michael Holquist, trans. Austin: University of Texas Press.

———. 1986. *Speech Genres and Other Late Essays.* Vern W. McGee, trans. Austin: University of Texas Press.

Barnes, Linda L. 1998. "The Psychologizing of Chinese Healing Practices in the United States." *Culture, Medicine, and Psychiatry* 22: 413–443.

———. 2003. "The Acupuncture Wars: The Professionalizing of American Acupuncture—A View from Massachusetts." *Medical Anthropology* 22, no. 3: 261–301. Available: http://www.acupunctureschools.us/The percent20Acupuncture percent20Wars.cfm, accessed March 8, 2007.

———. 2005a. *Needles, Herbs, Gods, and Ghosts: China, Healing, and the West to 1848.* Cambridge and London: Harvard University Press.

———. 2005b. "American Acupuncture and Efficacy: Meanings and Their Points of Insertion." *Medical Anthropology Quarterly* 19, no. 3: 239–266.

———. 2012. "A World of Chinese Medicine and Healing (Parts I and II)." In *Chinese Medicine and Healing: An Illustrated History,* ed. T. J. Hinrichs and Linda Barnes. Cambridge and London: Harvard University Press, 284–360.

Bauman, Richard. 2004. *A World of Others' Words: Cross-Cultural Perspectives on Intertextuality.* Malden, MA: Blackwell Publishing.

Bauman, Richard, and Charles Briggs. 2000. "Language Philosophy as Language Ideology: John Locke and Johann Gottfried Herder." In *Regimes of Language: Ideologies, Polities, and Identities,* ed. Paul V. Kroskrity. Santa Fe: School of American Research Press, 139–204.

———. 2003. *Voices of Modernity: Language Ideologies and the Politics of Inequality.* New York: Cambridge University Press.

Beagan, Brenda L. 2001. "'Even If I Don't Know What I'm Doing I Can Make it Look Like I Know What I'm Doing': Becoming A Doctor in the 1990's." *Canadian Review of Sociology and Anthropology* 38, no. 3: 275–292.

Beinfield, Harriet, and Efram Korngold. 1991. *Between Heaven and Earth: A Guide to Chinese Medicine.* New York: Ballantine Books.

———. 2001. "Centralism vs. Pluralism: Language, Authority, and Freedom in Chinese Medicine." *Clinical Acupuncture and Oriental Medicine* 2: 145–154.

Bellos, David. 2011. *Is That a Fish in Your Ear? Translation and the Meaning of Everything.* New York: Faber and Faber Inc.

Benksy, Dan, and Randall Barolet. 1990. *Chinese Herbal Medicine: Formulas & Strategies.* Seattle: Eastland Press.

Bensky, Dan, and Andrew Gamble (with Ted Kaptchuk). 1993. *Chinese Herbal Medicine: Materia Medica, Revised Edition.* Seattle: Eastland Press.

Bensky, Dan, Steven Clavey, and Erich Stöger (with Andrew Gamble). 2004. *Chinese Herbal Medicine: Materia Medica, Third Edition.* Seattle: Eastland Press.
Bensky, Dan, et al. 2006. "Toward a Working Methodology for Translating Chinese Medicine." *American Acupuncturist* 37: 14–15.
Bermann, Sandra, and Michael Wood, eds. 2005. *Nation, Language, and the Ethics of Translation.* Princeton and Oxford: Princeton University Press.
Bhabha, Homi. 1994. *The Location of Culture.* London and New York: Routledge.
Bosk, Charles L. 1979. *Forgive and Remember: Managing Medical Failure.* Chicago and London: University of Chicago Press.
Bourdieu, Pierre. 1991. *Language and Symbolic Power.* Gino Raymond and Matthew Adamson, trans. Cambridge, MA: Harvard University Press.
Boyarin, Jonathan, ed. 1993. *The Ethnography of Reading.* Berkeley: University of California Press.
Bruno, Gene. 2008. "AAAOM Delegates Attend Meeting of the World Federation of Chinese Medical Societies." *Acupuncture Today* 9, no. 2: 1. Available: www.acupuncturetoday.com/mpacms/at/article.php?id=31657, accessed May 3, 2009.
Brown, Michael F. 1997. *The Channeling Zone: American Spirituality in an Anxious Age.* Cambridge and London: Harvard University Press.
Buck, Charles. 2000. "On Terminology and Translation." *Journal of Chinese Medicine* 63: 38–42.
Buell, Paul D. 1989. "The Yin-shan Cheng-yao, a Sino-Uighur Dietary: Synopsis, Problems, Prospects." In *Approaches to Traditional Chinese Medical Literature: Proceedings of an International Symposium on Translation Methodologies and Terminologies,* ed. Paul U. Unschuld. Dordrecht: Kluwer Academic Publishers, 109–125.
———. 1998. "Chinese Medicine on the Gold Mountain." In *Disease and Medical Care in the Mountain West,* ed. Martha L. Hildreth and Bruce T. Moran. Reno and Las Vegas: University of Nevada Press, 95–139.
Burke, Adam. 2006. "The Naming of a Medicine." *American Acupuncturist* 37: 20–21.
Cao, Biyin. 2006. "Guanyu zhongyi yingyu fanyi jiben wenti he fazhan fangxiang de sikao (Pondering the problems and development of English translation for traditional Chinese medicine)." *Journal of Chinese Integrated Medicine* 4, no. 1: 108–110.
Capps, Lisa, and Elinor Ochs. 1995. *Constructing Panic: The Discourse of Agoraphobia.* Cambridge, MA: Harvard University Press.
———. 2002. "Cultivating Prayer." *In The Language of Turn and Sequence,* ed. Cecilia E. Ford, Barbara A. Fox, and Sandra A. Thompson. Oxford: Oxford University Press, 39–55.
Cassedy, James H. 1974. "Early Uses of Acupuncture in the United States." *Bulletin of the New York Academy of Medicine* 50, no. 8: 892–906.
Cassidy, Claire. 1998a. "Chinese Medicine Users in the United States, Part I: Utilization, Satisfaction, Medical Plurality." *Journal of Alternative and Complementary Medicine* 4, no. 1:17–27.
———. 1998b. "Chinese Medicine Users in the United States, Part II: Preferred Aspects of Care." *Journal of Alternative and Complementary Medicine* 4, no. 2: 189–202.
———. 2004. "What Does it Mean to Practice an Energy Medicine?" *Journal of Alternative and Complementary Medicine* 10, no. 1: 79–81.
Charon, Rita. 2001. "Narrative Medicine: A Model for Empathy, Reflection, Profession, and Trust." *JAMA* 286: 1897–1902.
Chase, Charles. 2006. "Asian Medical Nomenclature Debates." Paper presented at the Annual Meeting of the American Association of Oriental Medicine. Pheonix, October 19.

Chen, Ke-ji, and Ai-ping Lu. 2004. "Impressions on the Book 'On the Standard Nomenclature of Traditional Chinese Medicine' (by Professor Xie Zhu-fan)." *Chinese Journal of Integrated Medicine* 10, no. 1: 70–71.

Chen, Xinnong. 2005. *Chinese Acupuncture and Moxibustion, 2nd edition.* Beijing: Foreign Languages Press.

Clarke, J. J. 1997. *Oriental Enlightenment: The Encounter Between Asian and Western Thought.* London and New York: Routledge.

———. 2000. *The Tao of the West: Western Transformations of Daoist Thought.* London and New York: Routledge.

Clifford, James. 1997. *Routes: Travel and Translation in the Late Twentieth Century.* Cambridge and London: Harvard University Press.

Clift, Rebecca. 2006. "Indexing Stance: Reported Speech as an Interactional Evidential." *Journal of Sociolinguistics* 10, no. 5: 569–595.

Coleman, James William. 2001. *The New Buddhism: The Western Transformation of an Ancient Tradition.* New York: Oxford University Press.

Crapanzano, Vincent. 2011. "Metaphors of Legitimation/Legitimating Metaphors." Paper presented at the UCLA Center for Language, Interaction, and Culture Symposium on Legitimation Crises. Los Angeles, February 4.

Cronin, Michael. 2002. "The Empire Talks Back: Orality, Heteronomy, and the Cultural Turn in Interpretation Studies." In *Translation and Power,* ed. Maria Tymoczko and Edwin Gentzler. Amherst and Boston: University of Massachusetts Press, 45–62.

Csordas, Thomas J. 1994. "Introduction." In *Embodiment and Experience: The Existential Ground of Culture and Self,* ed. Thomas J. Csordas. Cambridge: Cambridge University Press, 1–26.

———. 2002. *Body/Meaning/Healing.* New York: Palgrave Macmillan.

———. 2008. "Intersubjectivity and Intercorporeality." *Subjectivity: International Journal of Critical Psychology* 22, no. 1: 110–121.

———. 2009. "Growing up Charismatic: Morality and Spirituality among Children in a Religious Community." *Ethos* 37, no. 4: 414–440.

Darnell, Regna. 2000. "Translation." *Journal of Linguistic Anthropology* 9, no. 1–2: 251–254.

Davenport, Beverly Ann. 2000. "Witnessing and the Medical Gaze: How Medical Students Learn to See at a Free Clinic for the Homeless." *Medical Anthropology Quarterly* 14, no. 3: 310–327.

Deadman, Peter. 2000. "Book Review: A Practical Dictionary of Chinese Medicine." *Journal of Chinese Medicine* 62: 54–56.

Deadman, Peter, and Mazin Al-Khafaji (with Kevin Baker). 2001. *A Manual of Acupuncture.* East Sussex: Journal of Chinese Medicine Publications.

Dechar, Lorie Eve. 2006. *Five Spirits: Alchemical Acupuncture for Psychological and Spiritual Healing.* New York: Chiron Publications/Lantern Books.

Ding, Weiyi. 2006. "Asian Medical Nomenclature Debates." Paper presented at the Annual Meeting of the American Association of Oriental Medicine. Phoenix, October 19.

Dobie, Sharon. 2007. "Reflections on a Well-Traveled Path: Self-Awareness, Mindful Practice, and Relationship-Centered Care as Foundations for Medical Education." *Academic Medicine* 82, no. 4: 422–427.

Duranti, Alessandro. 1993. "Intentions, Self, and Responsibility: An Essay in Samoan Ethnopragmatics." In *Responsibility and Evidence in Oral Discourse,* ed. Jane Hill and Judith T. Irvine. Cambridge: Cambridge University Press, 24–47.

Eckman, Peter. 1996. *In the Footsteps of the Yellow Emperor: Tracing the History of Traditional Acupuncture.* San Francisco: Cypress Book Company.

Eco, Umberto. 1979. *The Role of the Reader: Explorations in the Semiotics of Texts.* Bloomington: Indiana University Press.
Elder, William, et al. 2007. "Using Complementary and Alternative Medicine Curricular Elements to Foster Medical Student Self-Awareness." *Academic Medicine* 82, no. 10: 951–955.
Ellis, Andrew, Nigel Wiseman, and Ken Boss. 1989. *Grasping the Wind: An Exploration into the Meaning of Chinese Acupuncture Point Names.* Brookline: Paradigm Publications.
Emad, Mitra. 1998. "Feeling the Qi: Emergent Bodies and Disclosive Fields in American Appropriations of Acupuncture." Ph.D. dissertation, Department of Anthropology, Rice University.
———. 2006. "The Debate Over Chinese-Language Knowledge Among Culture Brokers of Acupuncture in America." *ETC: A Review of General Semantics* 63: 408–421.
———. In press. *Twirling the Needle: The Body as a Site for Translation in American Encounters with Acupuncture.* Albany, NY: SUNY Press.
English-Lueck, J. A. 1990. *Health in the New Age: A Study of California Holistic Health Practices.* Albuquerque: University of New Mexico Press.
Ergil, Marnae. 2001. "Considerations for the Translation of Traditional Chinese Medicine into English." Available: http://www.paradigm-pubs.com/refs/Translation.html, accessed November 17, 2005.
———. 2006. "Asian Medical Nomenclature Debates." Paper presented at the Annual Meeting of the American Association of Oriental Medicine. Phoenix, October 19.
Ergil, Marnae, and Kevin Ergil. 2006. "Issues Surrounding the Translation of Chinese Medical Texts into English." *American Acupuncturist* 37: 24–26.
Fairclough, Norman. 1992. *Discourse and Social Change.* Cambridge: Polity Press.
Farquhar, Judith. 1994. *Knowing Practice: The Clinical Encounter of Chinese Medicine.* Boulder: Westview Press.
Felt, Robert. 2000. "Reply to Charles Buck." *Journal of Chinese Medicine* 63: 44–46.
———. 2006a. "The Role of Standards in the Transmission of Chinese Medical Information." *American Acupuncturist* 37: 1820.
———. 2006b. "Readability in English language Chinese Medical Texts." Paper presented at the American Association of Oriental Medicine Meeting. Pheonix, October 19.
Flaws, Bob. 2000. "Letter to the Editor." *Journal of Chinese Medicine* 62: 52.
———. 2006a. "Arguments for the Adoption of a Standard Translational Terminology in the Study and Practice of Chinese Medicine." *American Acupuncturist* 37: 16–17, 27.
———. 2006b. "Asian Medical Nomenclature Debates." Paper presented at the Annual Meeting of the American Association of Oriental Medicine. Phoenix, October 19.
Flesch, Hannah. 2010. "A Foot in Both Worlds and Balance in Neither? Acupuncture, Education and Identity at a University of Natural Medicine in the United States." Ph.D. dissertation, Department of Anthropology, McMaster University.
Foley, William. 1997. *Anthropological Linguistics: An Introduction.* Oxford: Basil Blackwell.
Fox, Barbara. 2001. "Evidentiality: Authority, Responsibility, and Entitlement in English Conversation." *Journal of Linguistic Anthropology* 11, no. 2: 167–192.
Fratkin, Jake. 2006. "Asian Medical Nomenclature Debates." Paper presented at the Annual Meeting of the American Association of Oriental Medicine. Phoenix, October 19.
Friedrich, Hugo. 1992 [1965]. "On the Art of Translation." In *Theories of Translation: An Anthology of Essays from Dryden to Derrida,* ed. Rainer Schulte and John Biguenet. Chicago and London: University of Chicago Press, 11–16.
Furth, Charlotte. 1999. *A Flourishing Yin: Gender in China's Medical History, 960–1665.* Berkeley: University of California Press.

———. 2007a. "Introduction: Thinking with Cases." In *Thinking with Cases: Specialist Knowledge in Chinese Cultural History,* ed. Charlotte Furth, Judith T. Zeitlin, and Ping-chen Hsiung. Honolulu: University of Hawaii Press, 1–30.

———. 2007b. "Producing Medical Knowledge through Cases: History, Evidence, and Action." In *Thinking with Cases: Specialist Knowledge in Chinese Cultural History,* ed. Charlotte Furth, Judith T. Zeitlin, and Ping-chen Hsiung. Honolulu: University of Hawaii Press, 125–151.

Gadamer, Hans-Georg. 1981. *Reason in the Age of Science.* Frederick G. Lawrence trans. Cambridge and London: MIT Press.

———. 2004 [1975]. *Truth and Method.* Joel Weinsheimer and Donald G. Marshall, trans. London and New York: Continuum.

Gal, Susan. 1989. "Language and Political Economy." *Annual Review of Anthropology* 18: 345–367.

———. 2005. Language Ideologies Compared: Metaphors of Public and Private. *Journal of Linguistic Anthropology* 15: 23–37.

Garcia-Sanchez, Inmaculada, and Marjorie Faulstich Orellana. 2006. "The Construction of Moral and Social Identity in Immigrant Children's Narratives-in-Translation." *Linguistics and Education* 17: 209–239.

Given, Steve. 2006. "(CCAOM) Medical Nomenclature." *American Acupuncturist* 37: 26–27.

Goffman, Erving. 1974. *Frame Analysis: An Essay on the Organization of Experience.* Cambridge, MA: Harvard University Press.

Goldblatt, E. M., and W. H. Lee. 2010. "From Bench to Bedside: The Growing Use of Translational Research in Cancer Medicine." *American Journal of Translation Research* 2, no. 1: 1–18.

Goldstein, Michael. 1999. *Alternative Health Care: Medicine, Miracle, or Mirage?* Philadelphia: Temple University Press.

Good, Byron, and Mary-Jo Delvecchio-Good. 1981. "The Semantics of Medical Discourse." In *Sciences and Cultures,* ed. Everett Mendelsohn and Yehuda Elkana. Dordrecht: D. Reidel Publishing Company, 177–212.

———. 1993. "'Learning Medicine': The Constructing of Medical Knowledge at Harvard Medical School." In *Knowledge, Power, and Practice,* ed. Shirley Lindenbaum and Margaret Lock. Berkeley: University of California Press, 81–107.

———. 2000. "'Fiction' and 'Historicity' in Doctor's Stories: Social and Narrative Dimensions of Learning Medicine." In *Narrative and the Cultural Construction of Illness and Healing,* ed. Cheryl Mattingly and Linda Garro. Berkeley: University of California Press, 50–69.

Goodwin, Charles. 1994. "Professional Vision." *American Anthropologist* 96, no. 3: 606–633.

———. 1997. "The Blackness of Black: Color Categories as Situated Practice." In *Discourse, Tools, and Reasoning: Essays on Situated Cognition,* ed. Lauren B. Resnick, Roger Säljö, Clotilde Pontecorvo, and Barbara Burge. Berlin, Heidelberg, New York: Springer, 111–140.

Goodwin, Charles, and Alessandro Duranti. 1992. "Rethinking Context: An Introduction." In *Rethinking Context: Language as an Interactive Phenomenon,* ed. Charles Goodwin and Alessandro Duranti. Cambridge: Cambridge University Press, 1–42.

Graham-Pole, John. 2001. "'Physician, Heal Thyself': How Teaching Holistic Medicine Differs From Teaching CAM." *Academic Medicine* 76, no. 6: 662–664.

Greaves, D. 2002. "Reflections on a New Medical Cosmology." *Journal of Medical Ethics* 28: 81–85.

Grossman, Edith. 2010. *Why Translation Matters.* New Haven: Yale University Press.

Gumperz, John J., and Stephen C. Levinson, eds. 1996. *Rethinking Linguistic Relativity.* Cambridge: Cambridge University Press.

Hanks, William. 1989. "Text and Textuality." *Annual Review of Anthropology* 18: 95–127.

———. 1992. "The Indexical Ground of Deictic Reference." In *Rethinking Context: Language as an Interactive Phenomenon,* ed. Alessandro Duranti and Charles Goodwin, New York: Cambridge University Press, 43–76.

———. 2010. *Converting Words: Maya in the Age of the Cross.* Berkeley: University of California Press.

Hare, Martha L. 1993. "The Emergence of an Urban U.S. Chinese Medicine." *Medical Anthropology Quarterly* 7, no. 1: 30–49.

Hart, Roger. 1999. "Translating the Untranslatable: From Copula to Incommensurable Worlds." In *Tokens of Exchange: The Problem of Translation in Global Circulations,* ed. Lydia Liu. Durham: Duke University Press, 47–73.

Heelas, Paul. 1996. *The New Age Movement.* Malden, MA: Blackwell Publishing.

Heelas, Paul, et al. 2005. *The Spiritual Revolution: Why Religion is Giving Way to Spirituality.* Malden, MA: Blackwell.

Heinrich, Larissa N. 2008. *The Afterlife of Images: Translating the Pathological Body Between China and the West.* Durham: Duke University Press.

Heritage, John, and Douglas W. Maynard. 2006. *Communication in Medical Care: Interaction between Primary Care Physicians and Patients.* Cambridge: Cambridge University Press.

Heritage, John, and Geoffrey Raymond. 2005. "The Terms of Agreement: Indexing Epistemic Authority and Subordination in Assessment Sequences." *Social Psychology Quarterly* 68: 15–38.

Herzfeld, Michael. 2003. "The Unspeakable in Pursuit of the Ineffable: Representations of Untranslatability in Ethnographic Discourse." In *Translating Cultures,* ed. Paula G. Rubel and Abraham Rosman. Oxford and New York: Berg, 109–134.

Hill, Jane, and Judith T. Irvine. 1993. "Introduction." In *Responsibility and Evidence in Oral Discourse,* ed. Jane Hill and Judith T. Irvine. Cambridge: Cambridge University Press, 1–23.

Hinrichs, T. J., and Linda L. Barnes, eds. 2013. *Chinese Medicine and Healing: An Illustrated History.* Cambridge, MA, and London: The Belknap Press of Harvard University Press.

Ho, Evelyn Y. 2004. "'French Fries Have Too Much Huo Qi': An Ethnographic Study of the Discourse of Traditional Chinese Medicine." Ph.D. dissertation. Department of Communication Studies, University of Iowa.

———. 2006. "Behold the Power of Qi: The Importance of Qi in the Discourse of Acupuncture." *Research on Language and Social Interaction* 39, no. 4: 411–440.

———. 2007. "'Have You Seen Your Aura Lately?' Examining Boundary-work in Holistic Health Pamphlets." *Qualitative Health Research* 17, no. 1: 26–37.

Hobsbawm, Eric, and Terence Ranger. 1983. *The Invention of Tradition.* Cambridge: Cambridge University Press.

Hollan, Douglas. 2001. "Developments in Person-Centered Ethnography." In *The Psychology of Cultural Experience,* ed. Carmella C. Moore and Holly F. Mathews. Cambridge: Cambridge University Press, 48–67.

———. 2005. "Setting a New Standard: The Person-Centered Interviewing and Observation of Robert I. Levy." *Ethos* 33, no. 4: 459–466.

Holland, Dorothy C., et al. 1998. *Identity and Agency in Cultural Worlds.* Cambridge, MA.: Harvard University Press.

Hsu, Elisabeth. 1995. "The Manikin in Man: Culture Crossing and Creativity." In *Syncretism and the Commerce of Symbols*, ed. Göran Aijmer. Göteborg: The Institute for Advanced Studies in Social Anthropology, 156–204.

———. 1999. The *Transmission of Chinese Medicine*. Cambridge: Cambridge University Press.

———. 2010. *Pulse Diagnosis in Early Chinese Medicine: The Telling Touch*. Cambridge: Cambridge University Press.

Hui, Ka-kit, and Sonya E. Pritzker. 2007. "Terminology Standardization in Chinese Medicine: The Perspective From UCLA Center for East-West Medicine (Parts I and II)." *Chinese Journal of Integrated Medicine* 13, no. 1: 1–5, and 13, no. 2: 152–155.

Hui, Feng. 2009. "Different Languages, Different Cultures, Different Language Ideologies, Different Linguistic Models." *Journal of Multicultural Discourses* 4, no. 2: 151–164.

Irvine, Judith T. 1989. "When Talk Isn't Cheap: Language and Political Economy." *American Ethnologist* 16: 248–267.

———. 1996. "Shadow Conversations: The Indeterminacy of Participant Roles." In *Natural Histories of* Discourse, ed. Michael Silverstein and Greg Urban. Chicago: Univeristy of Chicago Press, 131–159.

Iser, Wolfgang. 1978. *The Act of Reading: A Theory of Aesthetic Response*. Baltimore: The Johns Hopkins University Press.

Jacob, Jeffrey H. 1996. *The Acupuncturist's Clinical Handbook*. New York: Integrative Wellness Inc.

Jarrett, Lonny S. 1998. *Nourishing Destiny: The Inner Tradition of Chinese Medicine*. Stockbridge, MA: Spirit Path Press.

Jakobson, Roman. 1966 [1959]. "On Linguistic Aspects of Translation." In *On Translation*, ed. Reuben A. Brower. New York: Oxford University Press, 232–239.

Jefferson, Gail. 1984. "Transcription Notation." In *Structures of Social Interaction*, ed. J. Maxwell Atkinson and John Heritage. New York: Cambridge University Press.

Jonas, Wayne B. 1998. "Alternative Medicine—Learning from the Past, Examining the Present, Advancing to the Future." *JAMA* 280, no. 18: 1616–1618.

Kao, Frederick F. 1992. "The Impact of Chinese Medicine on America." *American Journal of Chinese Medicine* 20, no. 1: 1–16.

Kaptchuk, Ted J. 2000. *The Web That Has No Weaver: Understanding Chinese Medicine (2nd Edition)*. New York: McGraw-Hill.

Kaptchuk, Ted J., and David Eisenberg. 1998. "The Persuasive Appeal of Alternative Medicine." *Annals of Internal Medicine* 129, no. 12: 1061–1065.

———. 2001. "Varieties of Healing.1: Medical Pluralism in the United States." *Annals of Internal Medicine* 135, no. 3: 189–195.

Karchmer, Eric. 2004. "Orientalizing the Body: Postcolonial Transformations in Chinese medicine." Ph.D. dissertation, Department of Anthropology, University of North Carolina at Chapel Hill.

———. 2010. "Chinese Medicine in Action: On the Postcoloniality of Medical Practice in China." *Medical Anthropology* 29, no. 3: 226–252.

Katz, Marian. 2011. "Chinese Medicine in the U.S.: Culture, Interaction, and the Construction of Patient-Centered Care." Ph.D. dissertation, Department of Sociology, University of California, Los Angeles.

Kendall, Donald E. 2002. *Dao of Chinese Medicine: Understanding an Ancient Healing Art*. Oxford: Oxford University Press.

Kershaw, Angela, and Gabriela Saldanha. 2013. "Introduction: Global Landscapes of Translation." *Translation Studies* 6, no. 2: 135–149.

Kligler, Benjamin, et al. 2004. "Core Competencies in Integrative Medicine for Medical School Curricula: A Proposal." *Academic Medicine* 79, no. 6: 521–531.

Konner, Melvin. 1987. *Becoming a Doctor: A Journey of Initiation in Medical School.* New York: G. P. Putnam's.

Kotarba, Joseph A. 1975. "American Acupuncturists: Entrepreneurs of Hope." *Urban Life* 4, no. 2: 148–177.

Kovacs, Jurgen. 1989. "Linguistic Reflections on the Translation of Chinese Medical Texts." In *Approaches to Traditional Chinese Medical Literature: Proceedings of an International Symposium on Translation Methodologies and Terminologies,* ed. Paul U. Unschuld. Dordrecht: Kluwer Academic Publishers, 85–95.

Kristeva, Julia. 1980. *Desire in Language: A Semiotic Approach to Literature and Art.* New York: Columbia University Press.

Kroskrity, Paul V. 2004. "Language Ideologies." In *Companion to Linguistic Anthropology,* ed. Alessandro Duranti. Malden, MA: Blackwell, 496–517.

Kuriyama, Shigehisa. 1994. "The Imagination of Winds and the Development of the Chinese Conception of the Body." In *Body, Subject, and Power in China,* ed. Angela Zito and Tani E. Barlow. Chicago and London: University of Chicago Press, 23–41.

———. 1999. *The Expressiveness of the Body and the Divergence of Greek and Chinese Medicine.* New York: Zone Books.

Larré, Claude, Jean Schatz, and Elisabeth Rochat de la Vallée. 1986. *Survey of Traditiona Chinese Medicine.* Sarah Elizabeth Stang, trans. Paris: Insitut Ricci and Columbia, MD: Traditional Acupuncture Institute.

Lao, Tzu. 1963. *Tao Te Ching* (DC Lau trans.). London: Penguin Books.

Le Blanc, Charles. 1995. "From Cosmology to Ontology through Resonance: A Chinese Interpretation of Reality." In *Beyond Textuality: Asceticism and Violence in Anthropological Interpretation,* ed. Gilles Bibeau and Ellen Corin. Berlin and New York: Mouton de Gruyter, 57–78.

Lei, Luo. 2004. "Zhongyi Yingyu Fanyi De Yuanze Chutan (A First Exploration of the Principles of the English Translation of Chinese Medicine)." *Journal of Chinese Integrated Medicine* 2, no. 3: 23–240.

Lei, Sean Hsiang-lin. 2002. "How Did Chinese Medicine Become Experiential? The Political Epistemology of Jingyan." *Positions* 10, no. 2: 333–364.

Levy, Robert, and Douglas W. Hollan. 1998. "Person Centered Interviewing and Observation." In *Handbook of Methods in Anthropology,* ed. H.R. Bernard. Walnut Creek: Altamira Press, 333–364.

Li, Shizhen, Hoc Ku Huynh, and G.M. Seifert, trans. 1985. *Pulse Diagnosis.* Brookline: Paradigm Publications.

Li, Zhaoguo. 2007. "Self-Criticism on the English Translation of Traditional Chinese Medicine." *Journal of Chinese Integrative Medicine* 5, no. 5: 598–603.

———. 2008a. "WHO xitaiqu ji 'shizhong lian' zhongyi mingci shuyu guoji biaozhun yanjiu: Zonglun bufen (Comparative Study on WHO Western Pacific Region and World Federation of Chinese Medical Societies International Standard Terminologies on Chinese Medicine: An Analysis of the General)." *Journal of Chinese Integrated Medicine* 6, no. 7: 761–765.

———. 2008b. "WHO xitaiqu ji 'shizhong lian' zhongyi mingci shuyu guoji biaozhun yanjiu: Yinyang xueshuo bufen (Comparative Study on WHO Western Pacific Region and World Federation of Chinese Medical Societies International Standard Terminologies on Chinese Medicine: An Analysis of the Yin-Yang Theory)." *Journal of Chinese Integrated Medicine* 6, no. 8: 878–880.

———. 2008c. "WHO xitaiqu ji 'shizhong lian' zhongyi mingci shuyu guoji biaozhun yanjiu: Wuxing xueshuo bufen (Comparative Study on WHO Western Pacific Region and World Federation of Chinese Medical Societies International Standard Terminologies on Chinese Medicine: An Analysis of the Five Elements Theory)." *Journal of Chinese Integrated Medicine* 6, no. 9: 983–986.

———. 2008d. "WHO xitaiqu ji 'shizhong lian' zhongyi mingci shuyu guoji biaozhun yanjiu: Jing, shen, qi, xue, jin, ye bufen (Comparative Study on WHO Western Pacific Region and World Federation of Chinese Medical Societies International Standard Terminologies on Chinese Medicine: An Analysis of the Essence, Spirit, Qi, Blood, Fluid, and Humor)." *Journal of Chinese Integrated Medicine* 6, no. 10: 1090–1093.

———. 2008e. "WHO xitaiqu ji 'shizhong lian' zhongyi mingci shuyu guoji biaozhun yanjiu: Zangfu bufen (Comparative Study on WHO Western Pacific Region and World Federation of Chinese Medical Societies International Standard Terminologies on Chinese Medicine: An Analysis of the Viscera)." *Journal of Chinese Integrated Medicine* 6, no. 11: 1200–1204.

———. 2008f. "WHO xitaiqu ji 'shizhong lian' zhongyi mingci shuyu guoji biaozhun yanjiu: Jingluo bufen (Comparative Study on WHO Western Pacific Region and World Federation of Chinese Medical Societies International Standard Terminologies on Chinese Medicine: An Analysis of the Meridians and Collatorals)." *Journal of Chinese Integrated Medicine* 6, no. 12: 1315–1317.

———. 2009a. "Comparative study on WHO Western Pacific Region and World Federation of Chinese Medical Societies International Standard Terminologies on Chinese Medicine: An Analysis of the Causes of Disease (Part I)." *Journal of Chinese Integrated Medicine* 7, no. 3: 284–287 [in English].

———. 2009b. "Comparative study on WHO Western Pacific Region and World Federation of Chinese Medical Societies International Standard Terminologies on Chinese Medicine: An Analysis of the Causes of Disease (Part II)." *Journal of Chinese Integrated Medicine* 7, no. 4: 383–388 [in English].

———. 2010. 1995 he 1997 zhongyi guojia biaozhun de yingyu fanyi wenti taolun (Discussion of the 1995 and 1997 National Standards for the English Translation of Chinese Medicine). *Journal of Chinese Integrative Medicine* 8, no. 11: 1090–1096.

Li, Zhaoguo, and Shulan Pan. 2009a. "Comparative Study on WHO Western Pacific Region and World Federation of Chinese Medical Societies International Standard Terminologies on Chinese Medicine: An Analysis of Body Constituents." *Journal of Chinese Integrated Medicine* 7, no. 1: 79–84 [in English].

———. 2009b. "Comparative Study on WHO Western Pacific Region and World Federation of Chinese Medical Societies International Standard Terminologies on Chinese Medicine: An Analysis of the Five Sensory Organs. *Journal of Chinese Integrated Medicine* 7, no. 2: 183–186 [in English].

———. 2009c. "Comparative Study on WHO Western Pacific Region and World Federation of Chinese Medical Societies International Standard Terminologies on Chinese Medicine: An Analysis of the Mechanism of Diseases (Part I)." *Journal of Chinese Integrated Medicine* 7, no. 5: 482–487 [in English].

Lianeri, Alexandra. 2002. "Translation and the Establishment of Liberal Democracy in Nineteenth-Century England: Constructing the Political as an Interpretive Act." In *Translation and Power*, ed. Maria Tymoczko and Edwin Gentzler. Amherst and Boston: University of Massachusetts Press, 1–24.

Light, Donald. 1980. *Becoming Psychiatrists: The Professional Transformation of Self.* New York and London: W.W. Norton and Company.

Lindholm, Charles. 2008. *Culture and Authenticity.* Malden, MA: Blackwell Publishing.

Liu, Lydia H. 1995. *Translingual Practice: Literature, National Culture, and Translated Modernity—China, 1900–1937.* Stanford: Stanford University Press.

———. 1999. "The Question of Meaning-Value in the Political Economy of the Sign." In *Tokens of Exchange: The Problem of Translation in Global Circulations,* ed. Lydia H. Liu. Durham: Duke University Press, 13–44.

Lo, Vivienne. 2001. "The Influence of Western Han Nurturing Life Literature on the Development of Acumoxa Therapy." In *Innovation in Chinese Medicine,* ed. Elisabeth Hsu. Cambridge: Cambridge University Press, 19–51.

———. 2009. "But is it [History of] Medicine? Twenty Years in the History of the Healing Arts of China." *Social History of Medicine* 22, no. 2: 283–303.

Lucy, John A. 1992. *Language Diversity and Thought: A Reformulation of the Linguistic Relativity Hypothesis.* Cambridge: Cambridge University Press.

Ma, Kanwen. 1989. "Classic Chinese Medical Literature in Contemporary China: Texts Selected for Modern Editions, and Problems Associated with This Work." In *Approaches to Traditional Chinese Medical Literature: Proceedings of an International Symposium on Translation Methodologies and Terminologies,* ed. Paul U. Unschuld. Dordrecht: Kluwer Academic Publishers, 7–17.

MacIntyre, Alasdair. 2007 [1981]. *After Virtue.* Notre Dame: University of Notre Dame Press.

Maciocia, Giovanni. n.d. "Note on the Translation of Chinese Terms." Available: http://www.giovanni-maciocia.com/pdf/terminology.pdf, accessed March 10, 2011.

———. 2000. "Reply to Charles Buck." *Journal of Chinese Medicine* 63: 50–52.

———. 2005. *The Foundations of Chinese Medicine: A Comprehensive Text for Acupuncturists and Herbalists (2nd edition).* London: Elsevier.

Malinowski, Bronislaw. 1978. *Coral gardens and their magic: A study of the methods of tilling the soil and of agricultural rites in the Trobriand Islands.* New York: Dover Publications.

McGuire, Katherine (with Debra Kantor). 1988. *Ritual Healing in Suburban America.* New Brunswick: Rutgers University Press.

Merleau-Ponty, Maurice. 1962 [2006]. *Phenomenology of Perception.* London and New York: Routledge.

Mitchell, Craig. 2006. "Asian Medical Nomenclature Debates." Paper presented at the Annual Meeting of the American Association of Oriental Medicine. Phoenix, October 19.

Mol, Annemarie. 2002. *The Body Multiple.* Durham: Duke University Press.

Montgomery, Kathryn. 2006. *How Doctors Think: Clinical Judgment and the Practice of Medicine.* Oxford: Oxford University Press.

Montgomery, Scott L. 2000. *Science in Translation: Movements of Knowledge Through Cultures and Time.* Chicago and London: Chicago University Press.

Narayan, Kirin. 1993. "How Native is a 'Native' Anthropologist?" *American Anthropologist* 95, no. 3: 671–686.

Nida, Eugene. 2000 [1964]. "Principles of Correspondence." In *The Translation Studies Reader,* ed. Lawrence Venuti. London and New York: Routledge, 126–140.

Nietzsche, Friedrich. 1992 [1882]. "On the Problem of Translation, Peter Mollenhauer, trans." In *Theories of Translation: An Anthology of Essays from Dryden to Derrida,* ed. Rainer Schulte and John Biguenet. Chicago and London: University of Chicago Press, 68–70.

Niu, Chuanyue. 2003. "Weishenme Yao Yanjiu Zhongyi Yingyu Fanyi (The Importance of Researching the English Translation of Chinese Medicine)." *Journal of Chinese Integrated Medicine* 1, no. 3: 239–240.

———. 2004. "Zailun zhongyi yingyu fanyi de yuanze (Further Discussion of the Principles of English Translation of Chinese Medicine)." *Journal of Chinese Integrated Medicine* 2, no. 3: 235–238.

———. 2005. "Zhongyi mingci shuyu guoji biaozhun zhunhua gongcheng zhengshi qidong (Program on International Standardization of Traditional Chinese Medicine Nomenclature Has Been Started)." *Journal of Chinese Integrated Medicine* 3, no. 1: 79–82.

———. 2006. "Mingyue songjian zhao, qingyong shishang liu: Zailun zhongyi yingyu fanyi jiqi guifanhua wenti (On Some Issues Concerning the Translation and Standardization of Traditional Chinese Medicine)." *Journal of Chinese Integrated Medicine* 4, no. 6: 657–660.

Novack, Dennis H., Ronald M. Epstein, and Randall H. Paulsen. 1999. "Toward Creating Physician—Healers: Fostering Medical Students' Self-awareness, Personal Growth, and Well-being." *Academic Medicine* 74, no. 5: 516–519.

Ochs, Elinor. 1984. "Language Acquisition and Socialization: Three Developmental Stories and Their Implications." In *Culture Theory: Essays on Mind, Self, and Emotion,* ed. Richard A. Schweder and Robert A. Levine. New York: Cambridge University Press, 276–320.

———. 2002. "Becoming a Speaker of Culture." In *Language Acquisition and Language Socialization: Ecological Perspectives,* ed. Claire Kramsch. New York: Continuum Press, 99–120.

———. 2010. "Semiotic Mediations of Experience." Paper presented at the Annual Meeting of the American Anthropological Association. New Orleans, November 19.

Ochs, Elinor, and Lisa Capps. 2001. *Living Narrative: Creating Lives in Everyday Storytelling.* Cambridge, MA: Harvard University Press.

Ochs, Elinor, and Sally Jacoby. 1995. "Co-construction: An Introduction." *Research on Language and Social Interaction* 28, no. 3: 171–183.

Ochs, Elinor, and Carolina Izquierdo. 2009. "Responsibility in Childhood: Three Developmental Trajectories." *Ethos* 37, no. 4: 391–413.

Ortega y Gasset, Jose. 1937 [1992]. "The Misery and the Splendor of Translation." Elizabeth Gamble Miller, trans. In *Theories of Translation: An Anthology of Essays from Dryden to Derrida,* ed. Rainer Schulte and John Biguenet. Chicago and London: University of Chicago Press, 93–112.

Parish, Steven M. 2008. *Subjectivity and Suffering in American Culture: Possible Selves.* New York: Palgrave Macmillan.

Paz, Octavio. 1992 [1971]. "Translation: Literature and Letters." Irene del Corral, trans. In *Theories of Translation: An Anthology of Essays from Dryden to Derrida,* ed. Rainer Schulte and John Biguenet. Chicago and London: University of Chicago Press, 152–162.

Pickering, Andrew. 1995. *The Mangle of Practice: Time, Agency, and Science.* Chicago and London: University of Chicago Press.

Pomerantz, Anita M. 1984. "Giving a Source or Basis: The Practice in Conversation of Telling 'How I Know.'" *Journal of Pragmatics* 8: 607–625.

Pordié, Laurent. 2012. "Branding Indian Aromatherapy. Trans-national Healthcare and the Making of Healing Practices." In *Authenticity, Best Practice, and the Evidence Mosaic: Integrating East Asian Medicines into Contemporary Healthcare,* ed. Volker Scheid and Hugh McPherson. London: Elsevier Press, 199–214.

Porkert, Manfred. 1974. *The Theoretical Foundations of Chinese Medicine: Systematic Correspondences.* Boston: MIT Press.

Poulet, Georges. 1969. "Phenomenology of Reading." *New Literary History* 1, no. 1: 53–68.

Pritzker, Sonya E. 2011a. "Standardization and Its Discontents: Four Snapshots in the Life of Language in Chinese Medicine." In *Authenticity, Best Practice, and the Evidence Mo-*

saic: Integrating East Asian Medicines into Contemporary Healthcare, ed. Volker Scheid and Hugh McPherson. London: Elsevier Press, 75–88.

———. 2011b. "The Part of Me that Wants to Grab: Embodied Experience and Living Translation in U.S. Chinese Medical Education." *Ethos* 39, no. 3: 395–413.

———. 2012a. "Living Translation in U.S. Chinese Medicine." *Language in Society* 41, no. 3: 343–364.

———. 2012b. "Standardization and its Discontents: Four Snapshots in the Life of Language in Chinese Medicine." In *Authenticity, Best Practice, and the Evidence Mosaic: Integrating East Asian Medicines into Contemporary Healthcare,* ed. Volker Scheid and Hugh McPherson. London: Elsevier Press, 75–88.

———. 2012c. "Transforming Self, World, Medicine: The Trend Toward Spiritualization in U.S. Chinese Medicine." In *Authenticity, Best Practice, and the Evidence Mosaic: Integrating East Asian Medicines into Contemporary Healthcare,* ed. Volker Scheid and Hugh McPherson. London: Elsevier Press, 203.

———. 2012d. "Textuality and Truth in U.S. Chinese Medicine Education." In *Chinese Medicine and Healing: An Illustrated History,* ed. T. J. Hinrichs and Linda Barnes. Cambridge and London: Harvard University Press, 318.

———. 2012e. "Translating the Essence of Healing: Inscription and Interdiscursivity in U.S. Translations of Chinese Medicine." *Linguistica Antverpiensia, New Series: Themes in Translation Studies* 11: 151–166.

———. In press. "Standardization and its Discontents: Translation, Tension, and the Life of Language in Contemporary Chinese Medicine." *East Asian Science and Technology Studies.*

Rabinow, Paul. 2008. *Marking Time: One the Anthropology of the Contemporary.* Princeton and Oxford: Princeton University Press.

Reiss, Katharina. 2000 [1971]. "Type, Kind and Individuality of Text: Decision Making in Translation." Susan Kitron, trans. In *The Translation Studies Reader,* ed. Lawrence Venuti. London and New York: Routledge, 160–171.

Ricœur, Paul. 1976. *Interpretation Theory: Discourse and the Surplus of Meaning.* Fort Worth: Texas Christian University Press.

Robinson, Douglas. 1991. *The Translator's Turn.* Baltimore: The Johns Hopkins University Press.

Rochat de la Vallée, Elisabeth. 2006. *A Study of Qi in Classical Texts.* King's Lynn: Monkey Press.

Roesler, Stéphanie. 2010. "Yves Bonnefoy's Metaphors on Translation." In *Thinking Through Translation with Metaphors,* ed. James St. André. Manchester, UK, and Kinderhook, NY: St. Jerome Publishing, 211–240.

Rogoff, Barbara. 1995. "Observing Sociocultural Activities on Three Planes: Participatory Appropriation, Guided Appropriation, and Apprenticeship." In *Sociocultural Studies of the Mind,* ed. James V. Wertsch, Pablo del Rio, and Amelia Alvarez. Cambridge: Cambridge University Press, 139–164.

Rosaldo, Renato. 1989. *Culture and Truth: The Remaking of Social Analysis.* Boston: Beacon Press.

Rosenberg, Z'ev. 2006. "A Position Paper on Terminology." *American Acupuncturist* 37: 28.

Ross, Anamaria Iosif. 2012. *The Anthropology of Alternative Medicine.* London and New York: Berg.

Rubel, Paula G., and Abraham Rosman, eds. 2003. *Translating Cultures.* Oxford and New York: Berg.

Sagli, Gry. 2010. "The Establishing of Chinese Medical Concepts in Norwegian Acupuncture Schools: The Cultural Translation of Jingluo ('Circulation Tracts')." *Anthropology and Medicine* 17, no. 3: 315–326.

Said, Edward. 1979. *Orientalism.* New York: Vintage Books.
Sapir, Edward. 1958 [1932]. "Cultural Anthropology and Psychiatry." In *Selected Writings of Edward Sapir,* ed. David G. Mandelbaum. Berkeley: University of California Press, 509–521.
Schegloff, Emanuel A. 1995. "Discourse as an Interactional Achievement III: The Omnirelevance of Action." *Research on Language and Social Interaction* 28, no. 3: 185–211.
Scheid, Volker. 2001. "Shaping Chinese Medicine: Two Case Studies From Contemporary China." In *Innovation in Chinese Medicine,* ed. Elisabeth Hsu. Cambridge: Cambridge University Press, 370–404.
———. 2002. *Chinese Medicine in Contemporary China.* Durham and London: Duke University Press.
———. 2007. *Currents of Tradition in Chinese Medicine: 1626–2006.* Seattle: Eastland Press.
Scheid, Volker, et al. 2009. *Chinese Herbal Medicine: Formulas & Strategies, 2nd ed.* Seattle: Eastland Press.
Schieffelin, Bambi. 2007. "Found in Translating: Reflexive Language across Time and Texts." In *Consequences of Contact: Language Ideologies and Social Transformation in Pacific Societies,* ed. Miki Makihara and Bambi B. Schieffelin. New York: Oxford University Press, 140–165.
———. 2008. "Tok Bokis, Tok Piksa: Translating Parables in Papua New Guinea." In *Social Lives in Language: Sociolinguistics and Multilingual Speech Communities,* ed. Miriam Meyerhoff and Naomi Nagy. Amsterdam: John Benjamins, 111–134.
Schieffelin, Bambi, and Ochs, Elinor. 1986. *Language Socialization across Cultures.* Cambridge and New York: Cambridge University Press.
Schliermacher, Friedrich. 1992 [1813]. "On the Different Methods of Translating." Waltraud Barscht, trans. In *Theories of Translation: An Anthology of Essays from Dryden to Derrida,* ed. Rainer Schulte and John Biguenet. Chicago and London: University of Chicago Press, 36–54.
Shen, Xiao Tian. 2006. "An Extra Thought about Nomenclature." *American Acupuncturist* 37: 12–13.
Shima, Miki. 2006. "Asian Medical Nomenclature Debates." *American Acupuncturist* 37: 811.
Shuman, Amy. 1993. "'Get Outa My Face': Entitlement and Authoritative Discourse." In *Responsibility and Evidence in Oral Discourse,* ed. Jane Hill and Judith T. Irvine. Cambridge: Cambridge University Press, 135–160.
Silverstein, Michael. 1979. "Language Structure and Linguistic Ideology." In *The Elements: A Parasession on Units and Levels,* ed. Paul R. Clyne, William Hanks, and Carol L. Hofbauer. Chicago: Chicago Linguistics Society, 193–247.
———. 1996. "The Secret Life of Texts." In *Natural Histories of Discourse,* ed. Michael Silverstein and Greg Urban. Chicago: University of Chicago Press, 81–105.
———. 2003. "Translation, Transduction, Transformation: Skating 'Glossando' on Thin Semiotic Ice." *In Translating Cultures,* ed. Paula G. Rubel and Abraham Rosman. Oxford and New York: Berg, 75–105.
Silverstein, Michael, and Greg Urban. 1996. "The Natural History of Discourse." In *Natural Histories of Discourse,* ed. Michael Silverstein and Greg Urban. Chicago: University of Chicago Press, 1–20.
Sinclair, Simon. 1997. *Making Doctors: An Institutional Apprenticeship.* Oxford and New York: Berg.
Sinn, Elizabeth. 2001. "Yan Fu." In *An Encyclopedia of Translation: Chinese-English, English-Chinese,* ed. Chan Sin-wai, and David E. Pollard. Hong Kong: Chinese University Press, 429–447.
Sivin, Nathan. 1987. *Traditional Medicine in Contemporary China.* Ann Arbor: Center for Chinese Studies, University of Michigan.

Spence, Jonathon D. 1990. *The Search for Modern China.* New York and London: W. W. Norton and Company.

Sterponi, Laura. 2004. "Reading as Involvement with Text." Ph.D. dissertation, Department of Applied Linguistics, University of California, Los Angeles.

———. 2007. "Reading as Involvement with Text: Insights from a Study of High Functioning Children with Autism." *Rivista Di Psicolinguisitca Applicata* 7, no. 3: 97–124.

Stivers, Tanya. 2012. "Language Socialization in Children's Medical Encounters." In *The Handbook of Language Socialization,* ed. Alessandro Duranti, Elinor Ochs, and Bambi Scheiffelin. Malden, MA: Wiley-Blackwell, 247–268.

Strauss, Sarah. 2005. *Positioning Yoga: Balancing Acts Across Cultures.* Oxford, New York: Berg.

Suh, Soyoung. 2013. "From the Common Cold to Incurable Diseases: The Korean Use of Shanghanlun, 1900–2012." Paper presented at the annual meeting of the Association for Asian Studies, San Diego, March 22.

Tambiah, Stanley J. 1990. *Magic, Science, Religion, and the Scope of Rationality.* Cambridge: Cambridge University Press.

Taylor, Charles. 1985. *Human Agency and Language: Philosophical Papers I.* Cambridge: Cambridge University Press.

———. 1989. *Sources of the Self: The Making of Modern Identity.* Cambridge, MA: Harvard University Press.

———. 1991. *The Ethics of Authenticity.* Cambridge, MA: Harvard University Press.

Taylor, Kimberly. 2001. "A New, Scientific, and Unified Medicine: Civil War in China and the New Acumoxa." In *Innovation in Chinese Medicine,* ed. Elisabeth Hsu. Cambridge: Cambridge University Press, 343–369.

———. 2004. "Divergent Interests and Cultivated Misunderstandings: The Influence of the West on Modern Chinese Medicine." *Social History of Medicine* 17, no. 1: 93–111.

Toury, Gideon. 2000 [1978]. "The Nature and Role of Norms in Translation." In *The Translation Studies Reader,* ed. Lawrence Venuti. London and New York: Routledge, 198–211.

Tymoczko, Maria, and Edwin Gentzler, eds. 2002. *Translation and Power.* Amherst and Boston: University of Michigan Press.

Unschuld, Paul U. 1985. *Medicine in China: A History of Ideas.* Berkeley: University of California Press.

———. 1989. *Approaches to Traditional Chinese Medical Literature: Proceedings of an International Symposium on Translation Methodologies and Terminologies.* Dordrecht: Kluwer Academic Publishers.

———. 2003. "The Spread of Traditional Chinese Medicine in the Western World: An Attempt at an Explanation of a Surprising Phenomenon." *Studies in the History of Natural Sciences* 22, no. 3: 215–222.

———. 2009. *What is Medicine? Western and Eastern Approaches to Healing.* Berkeley: University of California Press.

Van Hoy, Sarah Lee. 2010. "Authentic Traditions, Authentic Selves and Healing at the End of the World: An Auto-Ethnography of Chinese Medical Practices." Ph.D. dissertation, Department of Anthropology, University of Washington.

Van Wyke, Ben. 2010. "Imitating Bodies and Clothes: Refashioning the Western Conception of Translation." In *Thinking Through Translation with Metaphors,* ed. James St. André. Manchester, UK, and Kinderhook, NY: St. Jerome Publishing, 17–46.

Venuti, Lawrence. 1992. *Rethinking Translation: Discourse, Subjectivity, Ideology.* London: Routledge.

———. 2000. "Translation, Community, Utopia." In *The Translation Studies Reader,* ed. Lawrence Venuti. London and New York: Routledge, 468–488.

———. 2005. "Local Contingencies: Translation and National Identities." In *Nation, Language, and the Ethics of Translation,* ed. Sandra Berman and Michael Wood. Princeton and Oxford: Princeton University Press, 177–202.

Vygotsky, Lev S. 2004 "Thought and Word." In *The Essential Vygotsky,* ed. Robert W. Rieber and David K. Robinson. New York: Kluwer Academic, 65–110.

Wadensjö, Celia. 1998. *Interpreting as Interaction.* London and New York: Longman.

Wang, L. 1981. *Zhongguo yuyanxue shi* [*History of Chinese linguistics*]. Tyauan: Shanxi People's Press.

Wardwell, Walter I. 1994. "Alternative Medicine in the United States." *Social Science and Medicine* 38, no. 8: 1061–1068.

Weiss, Gail. 1999. *Body Images : Embodiment as Intercorporeality.* New York: Routledge.

Whorf, Benjamin. 1956 [1941]. *Language, Thought, and Reality: Selected Writings of Benjamin Lee Whorf.* Cambridge, MA: MIT Press.

Wikan, Uni. 1992. "Beyond the Words: The Power of Resonance." *American Ethnologist* 19, no. 3: 460–482.

Wilce, James. 2011. "Sacred Psychotherapy in the 'Age of Authenticity': Healing and Cultural Revivalism in Contemporary Finland." *Religions* 2: 566–589.

Wiseman, Nigel. n.d. "Westerners' Alternative Healthcare Values Eclipsing a Wealth of Knowledge." Available: http://www.paradigm-pubs.com/sites/www.paradigm-pubs.com/files/files/AltHeal.pdf. Accessed September 10, 2008.

———. 2000a. "Reply to Buck." *Journal of Chinese Medicine* 63: 38–42.

———. 2000b. "Reply to Buck and Maciocia." Available: http://www.paradigm-pubs.com/paradigm/refs/wiseman/JCMAnswer.pdf. Accessed 11/2005.

———. 2000c. "Translation of Chinese Medical Terminology: A Source-oriented Approach." Ph.D. dissertation, Department of Complementary Health Studies, Exeter University.

———. 2000d. "The Transmission and Reception of Chinese Medicine: Language, the Neglected Key." Paper presented at the Annual Pacific Symposium, San Diego, November 5.

———. 2001a. "The Extralinguistic Aspects of English Translation of Chinese Medical Terminology." Electronic document, available: http://www.paradigm-pubs.com/paradigm/refs/wiseman/Extralinguistics.pdf. Accessed November 15, 2005.

———. 2001b. "Reply to Beinfield and Korngold." *Clinical Acupuncture and Oriental Medicine* 2: 156–157.

———. 2002a. "Why the Fuss About Terminology?" Available (restricted access): F:\Papers\Dossier\3CHA2Fuss.doc, accessed November 3, 2005.

———. 2002b. "Against Anti-terminology." Available (restricted access): F:\Papers\Dossier\3CHA4Anti.doc, accessed November 3, 2005.

———. 2006. "English Translation of Chinese Medicine: Concerning the Use of Western Medical Terms to Represent Traditional Chinese Medical Concepts (Answer to Prof. Xie And His Colleagues)." *Chinese Journal of Integrated Medicine* 12, no. 3: 225–228.

Wiseman, Nigel, and Andrew Ellis. 1996. *Fundamentals of Chinese Medicine.* Brookline: Paradigm Publications.

Wiseman, Nigel, and Feng Ye. 1998. *A Practical Dictionary of Chinese Medicine.* Brookline: Paradigm Publications.

Wiseman, Nigel, and Paul Zmiewski. 1989. "Rectifying the Names: Suggestions for Standardizing Chinese Medical Terminology." In *Approaches to Traditional Chinese Medical Literature: Proceedings of an International Symposium on Translation Methodologies and Terminologies,* ed. Paul U. Unschuld. Dordrecht: Kluwer Academic Publishers, 55–64.

Wolfgram, Matthew. 2010. "Truth Claims and Disputes in Ayurveda Medical Science." *Journal of Linguistic Anthropology* 20, no. 1: 149–165.

Woolard, Kathryn A. 1985. "Language Variation and Cultural Hegemony: Towards an Integration of Sociolinguistic and Social Theory." *American Ethnologist* 12: 738–748.

———. 1998. "Introduction: Language Ideology as a Field of Inquiry." In *Language Ideologies: Practice and Theory,* ed. Bambi B. Scheiffelin, Kathryn A. Woolard, and Paul V. Kroskrity. New York and Oxford: Oxford University Press, 3–47.

World Federation of Chinese Medical Societies (WFCMS). 2007. *Basic Nomenclature in Traditional Chinese Medicine.* Beijing: People's Medical Publishing House.

World Health Organization–Western Pacific Region (WHO-WPR). *WHO International Standard Terminologies on Traditional Medicine in the Western Pacific Region* (Manila: WHO Library Cataloguing in Publication Data.

Wu, Jianguo. 2011. "Understanding Interdiscursivity: A Pragmatic Model." *Journal of Cambridge Studies* 6, no. 2: 95–115.

Xie, Zhufan. 2002a. "On Standard Nomenclature of Basic Chinese Medical Terms (II)." *Chinese Journal of Integrated Medicine* 8, no. 3: 231–234.

———. 2002b. "On Standard Nomenclature of Basic Chinese Medical Terms (IIIA)." *Chinese Journal of Integrated Medicine* 8, no. 4: 310–311.

———. 2003a. *On the Standard Nomenclature of Traditional Chinese Medicine.* Beijing: Foreign Languages Press.

———. 2003b. "On Standard Nomenclature of Basic Chinese Medical Terms (IV)." *Chinese Journal of Integrated Medicine* 9, no. 2: 148–151.

Xie, Zhu Fan, and P. White. 2005. "Comments on Nigel Wiseman's A Practical Dictionary of Chinese Medicine (I)—On the 'Word Forword' Literal Approach to Translation." *Chinese Journal of Integrated Medicine* 12, no. 4: 305–308.

———. 2006. "Comments on Nigel Wiseman's A Practical Dictionary of Chinese Medicine (II)—On the Use of Western Medical Terms to Express the Concepts of Traditional Chinese Medicine." *Chinese Journal of Integrated Medicine* 13, no. 1: 61–65.

Yafeh, Orit. 2007. "The Time in the Body: Cultural Construction of Femininity in Ultraorthodox Kindergartens for Girls." *Ethos* 36, no. 4: 516–553.

Yamada, Keiji. 1999. *Chugoku Igaku Wa Ikani Tsukuraretaka,* translated into Korean by Chŏn Sang-un and Yi Sŏng-gyu, Seoul: Saiŏnsŭbuksŭ (as cited by Suh 2013).

Yang, Xiaobin. 2007. "Jianping yifen yaopin shuomingshu de yingyi (Brief Comments on the English Translation of a Drug Direction)." *Journal of Chinese Integrated Medicine* 5, no. 3: 359–362.

Zhan, Mei. 2002. "The Worlding of Chinese Medicine: A Translocal Study of Knowledge, Identity, and Cultural Politics in China and the United States." Ph.D. dissertation, Department of Anthropology, Stanford University.

———. 2009. *Other-Wordly: Making Chinese Medicine Through Transnational Frames.* Durham and London: Duke University Press.

Zhang, Yanhua. 2007. *Transforming Emotions with Chinese Medicine: An Ethnographic Account from Contemporary China.* Albany: State University of New York Press.

Zhang, Yuhuan, and Ken Rose. 1995. *Who Can Ride the Dragon? An Exploration of the Cultural Roots of Traditional Chinese Medicine.* Brookline: Paradigm Publications.

Zhu, Jianping. 2002. *Zhongguo Yixueshi Yanjiu (Research into Chinese Medical History).* Beijing: Zhongyi Guji Chuban She.

Zhuo, Lian Shi. 2007. "Ganying Zhi Shen yu Zhenci Shoushen (Resonance to Treat the Spirit and Acupuncture to Guard the Spirit)." *Chinese Acupuncture and Moxibustion* 27, no. 5: 383–386.

Index